# *Step by Step*
# Regional Anesthesia

*System requirement:*

- **Windows XP or above**
- **Power DVD player (Software)**
- **Windows media player 10.0 version or above**
- **Quick time player version 6.5 or above**

*Accompanying CD ROM is playable only in Computer and not in CD player.*

Kindly wait for few seconds for CD to autorun. If it does not autorun then please follow the steps:

- Click on my computer
- Click the **drive labelled JAYPEE** and after opening the drive, kindly double click the file **Jaypee**

# *Step by Step*
# Regional Anesthesia

**Arun Kumar Paul**
BSc, MBBS, DA, MS (Anaesth.)
Ex-Prof of Anaesthesiology Medical College and Hospitals
Kolkata, West Bengal, India

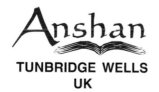

**TUNBRIDGE WELLS
UK**

**JAYPEE BROTHERS**
MEDICAL PUBLISHERS (P) LTD.
**New Delhi**

First published in the UK by

Anshan Ltd
**in 2008**
6 Newlands Road
Tunbridge Wells
Kent TN4 9AT, UK

Tel: +44 (0)1892 557767
Fax: +44 (0)1892 530358
E-mail: info@anshan.co.uk
www.anshan.co.uk

ISBN 13 978-1-848290-04-4

British Library Cataloguing in Publication Data
A catalogue record for this book is available from the British Library

Printed in India by Ajanta Offset & Packagings Ltd., New Delhi

*to*
*my loving wife, Kanyakumari*
*and*
*daughter, Sushmita*
*whose care and love*
*made this book possible*

# PREFACE

The present volume is a manual covering every relevant aspect of regional anaesthesia and analgesia particularly with the emphasis on the basic and practical applications. The intent is to provide a concise source of information in easy-to-understand style, so that conduction blocks can be practised confidently for better patient care.

A large number of line drawings and explanatory diagrams are incorporated to illustrate the commonly used techniques of conduction block including nerve blocks.

Materials have been consulted from the various authoritative books and works indicated in bibliography. I intend to express my indebtedness and appreciation to their authors and publishers. I also recommend them for further reading.

I am grateful to Shri JP Vij, Chairman and Managing Director of Jaypee Brothers Medical Publishers (P) Ltd. who actively cooperated during the entire project. I am thankful to Dr. PR Ghosh for kind assistance and Mr. Kajal Saha (Artist) for drawing the illustrations of the book.

I sincerely hope the volume will be a valuable guide book of regional anaesthesia/analgesia for all anaesthetists at all levels.

**Arun Kumar Paul**

# CONTENTS

# CHAPTER 1

# General Considerations

## BRIEF HISTORY

The term 'Regional Anaesthesia' was first used by Harvey Cushing in 1901 to describe pain relief by nerve block. Modern local anaesthesia started with the introduction of Cocaine into medical practice in 1984. It was introduced by Koller as a topical anaesthetic for the cornea. The first synthetic local anaesthetic, procaine was introduced by Einhorn in 1904, Lofgren and Lundqvist synthesized lignocaine in 1943. Lignocaine is the protolype local anaesthetic with which all other local anaesthetics are compared and judged.

A regional anaesthesia may be considered as the anaesthesia of an anatomical part of the body produced by the application of a chemical (local anaesthetic) agent capable to provide reversible conduction block of neural impulses associated with that part. Subsequent recovery from the effects of block is spontaneous and complete without any evidence of nerve damage.

## CLASSIFICATION

Regional anaesthesia is usually classified according to the site of application or administration of local anaesthetic to provide regional anaesthesia.

1. Topical or surface anaesthesia.
2. Local or infiltration anaesthesia
3. Intravenous regional anaesthesia (Bier's block)
4. Field block anaesthesia. It involves injecting local anaesthetic into the tissues about the periphery of the operative area.
5. Conduction anaesthesia. It is often designated as regional anaesthesia or nerve block anaesthesia. It is produced by injection of local anaesthetics along the course of nerve

plexus or nerves supplying the region of the body where the loss of sensation and of motor response is needed. It may be of three types:

(a) *Nerve blocks:* It is produced by injection of local anaesthetics near specific nerves to produce anaesthesia in areas innervated by the affected nerves.

(b) *Spinal analgesia:* It is produced by block of nerve roots in the subarachnoid space.

(c) *Epidural analgesia:* It is produced by block of nerve roots in the epidural space.

## Topical/Surface Anaesthesia

Here the local anaesthetic is applied over the skin surface or mucous membrane by spray, as in nose, mouth, or tracheo-bronchial tree, by spreading a local anaesthetic ointment, by instillation with syringe as into the urethra, by contact as with a saturated cotton pledget in nose or pharynx. Lignocaine (4%) spray may be applied topically on the pharynx and trachea before endotracheal intubation. Amethocaine is widely used to produce topical anaesthesia for bronchoscopy. The local anaesthetics which penetrate mucous membrane poorly (as procaine, chloroprocaine) are not suitable for topical anaesthesia.

EMLA cream (entectic mixture of lignocaine and prilocaine as an oil water emulsion) is applied to skin for at least 60 minutes to get a cutaneous anaesthesia.

## Local Infiltration Anaesthesia

This method is designed to produce sensory anaesthesia in the particular injected area without any attempt to block the particular nerves. Here the local anaesthetic is injected subcutaneously into the tissues to be cut as for placement of an intravenous catheter, paracentesis of the pleural or peritoneal cavities, lumbar puncture or suturing of tears and wounds.

### Plexus Blocks

Certain nerves are grouped together to form a plexus. If a plexus is blocked with the local anaesthetic, then several nerves can be blocked at the same time. Brachial plexus block is commonly employed to anaesthetize the upper extremity with a single injection of local anaesthetic.

## ADVANTAGES

1. The quality of analgesia and muscle relaxation are mostly satisfactory. Analgesia may continue even in early postoperative period.
2. Duration of analgesia may be adjusted with proper selection of local anaesthetic, its concentration, its volume and site of injection. Analgesia may be extended for prolonged period using either intermediate bolus injection or a continuous infusion.
3. Superior quality of analgesia may be provided for prolonged period with less haemodynamic disturbances.
4. Regional anaesthesia may provide satisfactory analgesia before, during and after surgery. It improves the patient's psychological state by abolishing the pain all the while.
5. Regional anaesthesia produces motor block causing profound muscular relaxation. It is advantageous for all surgical procedures.

6. In addition to sensory and motor block, regional anaesthesia provides autonomic block. As a result vasodilation may occur. It may help in the diagnosis and treatment of peripheral vascular diseases. Blood supply of skin flaps, amputation stumps, etc. improves and aids healing. It is particularly helpful in trauma surgery.

7. Adequate regional analgesia obviates the systemic ill effects of pain. It reduces the risk of postoperative complications and improves recovery. The systemic stress response to injury and surgery, the neuro-endocrine, metabolic and immunological responses to injury are minimum with regional anaesthesia and this helps to improve the surgical outcome significantly.

8. As the patients remain awake, the protective airway reflexes are intact all the while.

9. It can be used in outpatient clinic. It causes less physiologic disruption. Early discharge is possible.

10. Effective epidural analgesia protects the mother against the stress response to painful labour.

11. Regional anaesthesia for caesarean section decreases the risk of neonatal depression and maternal complications. Mother remains awake and can share the birth experience.

12. Regional anaesthesia needs minimal instrumentation and causes minimal physical and mental trauma.

## DISADVANTAGES

1. The technique needs full understanding of the topographical landmarks, nerve supply of the area, course of the related nerves, etc. It needs extra knowledge and skill regarding anatomy, physiology and pharmacology. Knowledge of surgical condition of disease is needed.

2. It is sometimes difficult and time consuming to provide neural blockade.
3. Drug allergy and toxicity may occur in some cases.
4. Some patients dislike injections.
5. Some patients dislike to remain awake during operation.
6. There may be failed or inadequate block.
7. Recovery time is uncontrollable.
8. In cases with spinal/epidural anaesthesia there may be difficulty in voiding, back pain, post-dural puncture headache and so on.
9. Decrease in blood pressure may occur due to peripheral sympathetic nervous system block by regional anaesthesia particularly in hypovolaemic patients.
10. Non-cooperative patients such as acutely intoxicated and agitated patients are not fit for regional anaesthesia.
11. Lack of practice may increase the rate of failures of block.

## INDICATIONS

1. Anaesthesia
2. Postoperative analgesia
3. Diagnosis of chronic pain syndromes
4. Treatment of chronic pain syndromes

Besides the common popular indications to provide anaesthesia and postoperative analgesia, diagnosis and treatment of chronic pain syndromes are most important. Differential nerve blocks are often used to distinguish placebo, sympathetic and somatic sensory sources of pain. Pain is said to be psychogenic when relief is obtained by placebo injection in subarachnoid space. When relief is obtained with 0.2% procaine injection, the pain is due to sympathetic nervous symptom pathway. If pain persists after 1% procaine injection, pain seems to be due to more central origin or pshychogenic. Stellate ganglion block or lumbar sympathetic block is also being used to detect the sympathetic nervous system origin of pain.

Therapeutic nerve blocks are also being used with local anaesthetics, neurolytic agents or neuroaxial placement of opioids.

The other indications of regional anaesthesia may also include –

1. *Patient preference:* Patient wants to remain awake during surgery. Mother may want to share the birth experience.
2. *Prolonged surgery:* Many patients may feel very tiresome and uncomfortable to lie still for more than an hour or two.
3. In some cases where general anaesthesia is contraindicated and somewhat hazardous due to physical or metabolic derangement, regional anaesthesia may confer benefits of their own. But it should be noted that regional anaesthesia is not always simply alternative to general anaesthesia and it should be judged against merits demerits ratio.

## CONTRAINDICATIONS TO REGIONAL ANAESTHESIA

The contraindications are mostly relative. As there are so many methods, one can modify the technique and choose the site of injection and local anaesthetic for better patient care.

All patients should be prepared and well investigated for major operations whether it is scheduled for general or regional anaesthesia. It does not mean that regional anaesthesia needs less investigations and preparation and it is easy and less demanding bypass to general anaesthesia. Pathophysiological disturbances should always be corrected prior general or regional anaesthesia.

However, the relative contraindications may be as follows:

1. Refusal. Patient wants to loose his consciousness during operation.
2. Patients with psychological or psychiatric disturbances.
3. Patients with coagulation disorders.
4. Presence of infection at the site of injection.
5. Trauma/injury/burns over the site of injection.
6. Patients with metabolic disorders not adequately treated.
7. Pre-existing neurological deficit.
8. Where sterility of the equipment is not guaranteed.
9. Where basic resuscitative equipment and drugs are not available.
10. Where proper valid consent is not present.
11. Lack of knowledge and practice on the part of anaesthetist.

## GENERAL PRINCIPLES

1. Anaesthetist should have a knowledge of the history of the disease concerned and his pathophysiological status.
2. Anaesthetist should be properly trained and have adequate knowledge and skill to tackle the case even when the complications arise.
3. The patient should be well informed about the technique and discuss all merits and demerits.
4. Patient should give proper valid consent.

5. Proper psychic preparation of the patient is needed. Patient should be reassured and complete confidence is essential. Adequate and complete explanation is helpful.

6. Proper preparation for anaesthesia is always needed.

7. Pharmacologic premedication is always beneficial.

8. Surgical rules:

   (a) Regional anaesthesia technique should be regarded as surgical procedure. Aseptic precautions are essential. Anaesthetist should scrub, be properly gowned and gloved.

   (b) All instruments should be sterilised.

   (c) Skin preparation on the site of injection should be adequate.

   (d) Proper ventilation, lighting arrangements, asepsis, good operating table, sterilised instrument tray should be fool proof.

   (e) Emergency resuscitation equipment, drugs, defibrillator, pacemaker, etc. should be kept ready.

   (f) General anaesthesia may be needed in some failed cases, thus anaesthesia machine, drugs and equipment should always be there. Oxygen supply should be available.

   (g) Injection site should be aseptically drapped.

   (h) Avoid injection to infected site.

9. Anaesthetist should know the basic **pharmacological aspects** of the local anaesthetic drugs.

   (a) Local anaesthetic vails should be sterile and kept in aseptic instrument tray.

   (b) Syringe, needle, lumbar puncture needle, epidural (Tuhoy needle), catheters should be kept in sterile condition.

(c) Dose should be calculated properly and least amount of drug should be used.

(d) Least toxic drug should be used.

(e) Dose and strength and volume should be judged according to individual patient, site of operation, approximate duration of operation, etc. Safe maximum dose of the concerned drug should be kept in mind.

(f) Potentiation problems. Spread of drugs, metabolism of drugs, onset of action and duration of anaesthesia should always be considered during selection of local anaesthetics.

(g) Complications, systemic toxicity, hypersensitivity reactions, if arise should be promptly diagnosed and tackled accordingly.

10. Success of regional anaesthesia mostly depends on depositing the local anaesthetic solution accurately on a particular space to block the specified nerves. Techniques are mostly blind and depend on anatomical landmarks. Some landmarks either superficial or deep are being used. Superficial landmarks include skin measurements, bony prominences, arterial pulsations, fixed visual points, etc. Deep landmarks are sensations of the advancing needle point into fascial planes, ligaments, deep tendons, bony structures, foramina, etc.

(a) Measurements should always be accurate with the help of a ruler. Special marking pencils may be used.

(b) Deep landmarks should be identified gently and accurately with due sensation of touch of progressing the needle point. Better identification of the tissue and of depth is acquired by practice.

(c) Avoid paraesthesia deliberately. However, if paraesthesia is obtained the needle should be withdrawn a few mm before injection.

(d) Never inject directly to nerve trunk.

(e) Needle should be gently directed towards bone. Note that the periosteum is extremely sensitive.

(f) Radiologic help is often useful for diagnosis and therapeutic nerve blocks for accurate placement of needles and/or verification of needle position at the time of injection of local anaesthetics.

(g) Use of nerve stimulation may help to locate the nerve.

11. Technical skill is most important for the outcome of the procedure.

(a) Equipment for regional anaesthesia include proper size syringes and a set of needles. These should be tested beforehand and sterilised properly. Chemical sterilisation is not recommended.

(b) Intradermal wheal is essential to make the injection painfree.

(c) Local anaesthetic solution should be fresh.

(d) Multiple puncture for injection should be avoided.

(e) Site of injection should be accurate.

(f) Aspiration test is mandatory before actual injection of the drug. After the first aspiration test, the needle should be rotated in $180°$ and repeat the test.

(g) Injection should be given gently. It should not be sudden and not excessively rapid.

(h) Avoid infected or inflamed site of injection.

(i) Allow the surgeon to start operation after anaesthesia is established. Sufficient time should be given to establish the complete block.

## CAUSES OF FAILURE OF BLOCKS

1. *Variations of nerve anatomy:* Blind technique may miss the site of nerve and block.
2. *Variations of landmark anatomy:* Distorted landmarks may lead to failure of block.
3. *Lack of knowledge and skill of the anaesthetist:* Adequate knowledge of anatomy, physiology and pharmacology is needed. Dose, strength and volume of local anaesthetic solution should be accurately judged.
4. Lack of practice may lead to error and hence failure of block.
5. Diagnostic and therapeutic nerve blocks for chronic pain syndromes need careful evaluation of pain. Psychic and emotional factors should be borne in mind.

• Some patients may need general anaesthesia along with regional anaesthesia.

1. Children may receive regional anaesthesia after induction of general anaesthesia. Risk of neural damage becomes less.
2. Some blocks like intercostal, interpleural, femoral, sciatic nerve blocks are usually performed after induction of general anaesthesia.
3. Patient intends to remain unconscious even when he prefers regional anaesthesia.
4. Prolonged lengthy surgical procedures.
5. To obviate tourniquet pain.
6. If surgery causes reflex stimuli outside the area of regional anaesthesia, general anaesthesia may be helpful.
7. If the patient becomes non-cooperative during the course of surgery, general anaesthesia may have be combined.
8. Surgical procedures like amputations, cancer surgery, etc. may need combined general and regional anaesthesia for better outcome.

# Pharmacology
of Local
Anaesthetics

## INTRODUCTION

Local anaesthetics produce reversible interruption to the conduction of neural impulses by their effect on the sodium channels of neurons. They interrupt transmission of autonomic, sensory and motor neuronal impulses resulting autonomic nervous system block, sensory anaesthesia and skeletal muscle paralysis in the part innervated by the affected nerves. Subsequent recovery is spontaneous and complete.

Following administration of a local anaesthetic drug into the tissues it is metabolised by local hydrolysis as in case of ester local anaesthetics, bound to protein and passes away into circulation. Of the remaining molecules, tissue pH and each drug pKa dictate the ratio of the drug existing as an uncharged base and as a positively charged ion. The free base form of the drug penetrates various tissue layers to reach the nerve axon and the cationic form acts on the sodium channel. Local anaesthetics drugs depress sodium conductance through sodium channels by stabilising and maintaining sodium channels in the inactivated closed states by binding to specific receptors present in the inner portion of sodium channels. These also prevent changes in sodium permeability by obstructing sodium channels near their external openings. Thus, it slows the rate of depolarisation as a result the threshold potential is not reached and the action potential is not propagated along the nerve membrane. Ion gradients and resting transmembrane potentials or threshold potentials remain unaltered. But the rate and amplitude of depolarisation are consequently decreased.

## USE DEPENDENT BLOCK

Most of the local anaesthetic drugs possess **use-dependence.** More the channels are opened the greater will be the block. Here the anaesthetic molecules are able to reach the site of action more easily when the channels are in activated-open states. Repetitive artificial depolarisation of a nerve causes the sodium channels in open state more frequently recruits more of them and maintains open state for longer period. Drug uptake by the sodium channel is also enhanced. Only the local anaesthetic cation can produce frequency dependent block, but not the unionised base.

## MINIMUM BLOCKING CONCENTRATION

This is defined as the minimum concentration of a local anaesthetic drug that will prevent impulse conduction *in vitro* in a specific nerve within a specific time. This is not much significant in clinical anaesthesia. But it may be of value when comparing the potencies of individual drugs.

## DIFFERENTIAL NEURAL BLOCK

Nerves differ to their sensitivity to local anaesthetic agents according to the fibre diameter, presence or absence of myelin and function. Differential effects are mostly observed during the onset of block gradually progressing in the following order:

(a) Vasodilatation ($\beta$ fibres)
(b) Loss of pain and temperature (C and A$\delta$ fibres)
(c) Loss of muscle spindle reflex (A$\delta$ fibres)
(d) Loss of motor and pressure (A$\beta$ fibres)
(e) Loss of large motor and proprioception (A$\alpha$ fibres)

- Function of nerve fibres:
  - $A\alpha$ (10-20 μm): motor, proprioception
  - $A\beta$ (5-12 μm): touch, pressure
  - $A\gamma$ (3-6 μm): motor to muscle spindle
  - $A\delta$ (2-5 μm): pain, touch, temperature
  - B (less than 3 μm): preganglionic autonomic
  - C (0.2 to 1.4 μm): postganglionic autonomic

In general, they block nerve conduction in small diameter nerve fibres more easily than in large fibres. The small $A\delta$ and unmyelinated C fibres are most sensitive to local anaesthetics in comparison to $A\beta$ and large motor fibres and these are most resistant. It is also apparent that the nerve fibres located close to the nerve surface and exposed to the local anaesthetic solution are more easily and quickly blocked.

Myelination offers resistance to the effects of local anaesthetics. The myelin sheath is devoid of sodium channels. Local anaesthetic works better in an area of high sodium channel density present at the nodes of Ranvier of the myelin sheath. Thus, a large nerve fibre with long internodal distance will need larger quantity of drug to produce satisfactory block in comparison to small nerve fibre with short internodal distance or unmyelinated nerve fibre.

## GENERAL PHARMACOLOGY

Local anaesthetics consist of an aromatic ring and a carbon chain bearing amino group. These two are joined either by an ester or an amide link. Thus, local anaesthetics are popularly classified as amino-esters and amino-amides.

1. *Ester local anaesthetics:* Procaine, cocaine, chloro-procaine, tetracaine.

2. *Amide local anaesthetics:* lignocaine, prilocaine, mepivacaine, bupivacaine, etidocaine, ropivacaine.

These two groups of drugs differ in relation to the site of metabolism, potential to produce allergic reactions and stability in solution. The ester drugs are metabolised by plasma esterase, are unstable in solution and their allergic reactions are relatively common. The amide drugs undergo hepatic enzymatic metabolism, degraded by hepatic endoplasmic reticulum involving N-deacylation and subsequent hydrolysis. These are stable and their allergic reactions are extremely rare.

## LIPID SOLUBILITY

Anaesthetic potency depends on lipid solubility of the local anaesthetic. The more lipid soluble drug molecules have the capacity to penetrate the neural membrane more readily and thus they possess greater potency. Lipid-water partition coefficient of the local anaesthetic is directly related to the minimum concentration needed for conduction block. The greater the partition coefficient the greater the lipid solubility. Drugs with partition coefficient less than 1 require concentration 2 to 3%, with coefficients of 1 to 3 require 1 to 2% and with coefficients of more than 4 require 0.25 to 0.5% concentration for conduction block.

## pKa

The pKa of local anaesthetic determines the amount of unionised drug available for diffusion across the lipophilic nerve membrane and subsequently the amount of ionised drug available for sodium channel blocking. The pKa is the pH at which the one-half the drug is unionised free base and the other half is cation.

## PROTEIN BINDING

Protein binding of local anaesthetic determines the duration of action of local anaesthesia. Drugs with low protein binding have a rapid onset of action and short duration of action. Drugs with high protein binding have a slow onset and long duration of effect. As for example, bupivacaine, etidocaine and ropivacaine are highly protein bound about 90% or more. Local anaesthetic may bind to tissue proteins at perineural sites (protein component of nerve membrane). They also bind to alpha glycoprotein and albumin in plasma. High affinity for tissue and plasma proteins may be associated with high affinity for the sodium channel binding protein.

## EFFECT ON BLOOD VESSELS

Most local anaesthetics are vasodilators. The vasodilator actions of the drugs influence their efficacy and duration of action. Following injection of local anaesthetic drug, some is taken up by neural tissue and some part is taken away by the blood perfused in the adjoining area. Cocaine causes vasoconstriction due to block of neural uptake of noradrenaline.

Vasoconstrictor drugs particularly adrenaline may be added to local anaesthetic drug to reduce absorption. This may cause more effective and longer duration of anaesthesia. It improves the quality of block. It also reduces the rate of rise and peak blood levels of local anaesthetics and thereby reduces the risk of systemic toxicity.

Adrenaline is the vasoconstrictor of choice in local anaesthetics in a concentration of 5 µg/ml (1: 200000) to a maximum dose of 200 mg. Larger doses may not give additional advantage, but carry the risk of cardiac arrhythmias.

Addition of adrenaline to local anaesthetic solution is not advised in following conditions:

1. Myocardial ischaemia
2. Cardiac dysrhythmia
3. Hypertensive patients
4. Utero-placental insufficiency
5. Intravenous regional anaesthesia
6. On the site lacking collateral blood flow as in digits, penis, etc.

## ROLE OF ALKALINE pH ADJUSTMENT ON LOCAL ANAESTHETIC BLOCK

Bicarbonate is often added to local anaesthetic solution to reduce the onset time particularly in epidural block. It may increase the amount of drug in the uncharged base form which may increase diffusion through nerve sheaths and nerve membranes.

## IDEAL CHARACTERISTICS OF LOCAL ANAESTHETICS

1. Potent, reliable, safe
2. Effective in low concentration
3. Rapid onset of action
4. Long duration of action
5. Low systemic toxicity
6. Nonirritant, no tissue/nerve damage

7. Reversible action
8. Can be easily sterilised
9. Cheap, easily available in different strengths.

## ADVERSE EFFECTS

These are mostly due to systemic toxicity, local toxicity, hypersensitivity and agent specific effects.

## SYSTEMIC TOXICITY

This is mostly due to excess plasma concentration of the drug. Various factors may influence the toxicity. These may include type of the drug, total dose and concentration of the drug, rate of rise of plasma levels, drug overdose (absolute or relative), inadvertent intravascular injection, vascularity of local tissue, presence of vasoconstrictors like adrenaline, physical condition of the patient, any liver or kidney disease and so on. Total fraction of unbound drug in circulation is also a major factor.

The toxic effects of a local anaesthetic initially include tinnitus, perioral and tongue numbness, confusion, light headedness, visual disturbances and so on. Then it is followed by excitation phase manifested by anxiety, restlessness, muscle twitching and even grand mal seizures. This phase is due to blockade of inhibitory pathways allowing facilitatory neurons to discharge without the normal negative input.

Then there is depression phase causing unconsciousness, generalised central nervous system depression and even respiratory arrest.

During this process, there is excitatory phase of medulla (tachycardia, hypertension, tachypnoea, nausea/vomiting) followed by medullary depression (bradycardia, apnoea, hypotension, coma, cardiac arrest).

Cardiovascular effects may include depressive phase (bradycardia, hypotension, sinus arrest) and excitatory phase (supraventricular tachycardia, ventricular fibrillation). These may be associated with hypoxia, acidosis and hyperkalaemia. Allergic responses may also be there.

*Treatment of toxicity involves:*
1. Immediate stoppage of drug injection
2. Administration of oxygen
3. Maintenance of airway
4. Artificial ventilation
5. IV diazepam 0.1 mg/kg to treat convulsion.
6. Specific inotropes or antiarrhythmic drug to combat cardiovascular toxicity.
7. General supportive measures/care.
   IV infusion, IV vasopressors
- Prevention of toxicity should always be attempted with the following:
1. Anaesthetist should have adequate skill and knowledge.
2. Dose should be accurately calculated and given gently.
3. Constant monitoring during anaesthesia is essential
4. Intravascular injection should be avoided. Repeated aspiration test should be done before injection.
5. Resuscitative drugs and equipment should be readily available.
6. Early diagnosis and immediate treatment are most essential.

## LOCAL TISSUE TOXICITY

It may occur on the tissues at the site of injection. Localised nerve damage is extremely rare. Prolonged exposure of nerves to higher concentrations may cause prolonged sensorimotor deficits particularly following spinal block with hyperbaric lignocaine through fine catheters. Myotoxicity may occur following IM injection particularly with cocaine.

## HYPERSENSITIVITY REACTIONS

Some patients may have allergic response manifested by erythema, rash, urticaria, oedema, bronchospasm and hypotension. Laryngeal oedema, pulmonary oedema, respiratory distress and cardiac arrhythmias can also occur. It is common following use of ester group of local anaesthetics as these are metabolised to parabenzoic acid which may cause allergy. The amide group of local anaesthetics are mostly safe, but its preservative containing methylparaben and sodium metabisulphite, an antioxidant may cause allergic responses. Prevention may be tried with the following:

1. Avoid the specific drug in patients with past history of allergic reactions.
2. Test doses (intradermal) may be given to detect any allergic response before actual injection.
3. Preservative free amide local anaesthetic may be used.

*Treatment of hypersensitivity reactions*

1. Oxygen
2. IV fluid
3. Adrenaline, hydrocortisone

4. *Antihistaminics:* Diphenhydramine
5. *Bronchodilators:* Albuterol inhalation
6. Specific therapy according to manifestations.

## Drug Specific

Prilocaine may induce methemoglobinemia due to accumulation of a metabolite 6-hydroxytoluidine and is mostly dose related.

Cocaine may cause dependence due to cerebral stimulation and euphoric effects.

Lignocaine may cause cauda equina syndrome following spinal block by using microspinal catheters.

Chloroprocaine causes neurological damage and it should not be used in subarachnoid block and intravenous regional anaesthesia. It is mostly due to the preservative sodium metabisulphite.

## *Uses of Local Anaesthetics*

1. Regional anaesthesia
2. IV lignocaine –
   (a) to prevent and treat ventricular dysrhythmias.
   (b) to attenuate pressor responses of tracheal intubation.
   (c) to prevent and treat the rise in intracranial pressure during tracheal intubation.
   (d) to minimise cough reflex during laryngoscopy and endotracheal intubation.
- Recommended safe maximum single dose of some common local anaesthetics in adults:

| Drug | mg/kg without adrenaline | mg/kg with adrenaline |
|---|---|---|
| Lignocaine | 4 | 7 |
| Mepivacaine | 4 | 7 |
| Bupivacaine | 2.5 | 3.2 |
| Etidocaine | 6 | 8 |
| Prilocaine | 7 | 8.5 |
| Chloroprocaine | 11 | 14 |

- Vasoconstrictors are often mixed with local anaesthetic solution with the aim to reduce the risk of systemic toxicity and to extend the duration of block. Vasoconstriction helps to limit the absorption of drugs and improves the quality of block. Adrenaline is being widely used in concentration of 5 μg/ml (1 : 200,000) to a maximum dose 200 μg. Larger doses may not give further benefit and may carry the risk of cardiac arrhythmias. Other drugs like phenylephrine, octapressin, noradrenaline are not much popular as these may not confer any particular advantage.

## COMMONLY USED DRUGS

Large number of drugs are available, but the most commonly used local anaesthetics are lignocaine and bupivacaine. Lignocaine is recommended due to its short or moderate duration of effect. But bupivacaine is chosen when the longer duration of block is required. However, prilocaine, ropivacaine, and other drugs are also being used.

### Lignocaine

Lignocaine is the standard local anaesthetic agent most widely used and all others are compared with it. It is of moderate potency and duration of effect and there is rather slow onset of action. Adrenaline is used with it to prolong its effect and reduce its systemic toxicity. The maximum safe dose by single injection is 300 mg and may be increased to 500 mg with the addition of adrenaline. Duration of anaesthesia following infiltration is about 1 hour, but may be increased to about 2 hours when mixed with adrenaline. The concentration of adrenaline in lignocaine solution is 1 in 200000 dilution.

It is used for topical analgesia, infiltration anaesthesia, peripheral nerve block, intravenous regional anaesthesia, spinal, epidural and caudal analgesia. It is available as injectable hydrochloride salt solutions in different strengths ranging from 0.5 to 2%. It is available in 4% viscous, gel and metered aerosol forms, some solutions are with adrenaline 5 µg/ml. Sodium chloride is added to these solution to achieve isotonicity. The preservatives are sodium metabisulphite and methyl parahydroxybenzoate.

It is also a constituent of EMLA cream. Entectic mixture of local anaesthetics is a mixture of lignocaine and prilocaine as an oil-water emulsion and widely used for cutaneous anaesthesia.

Lignocaine is also used as an antiarrhythmic agent by continuous IV infusion. It has been used in the management of neonatal convulsions, chronic pain syndromes and as a parenteral analgesic.

## Prilocaine

It has medium onset of action and moderate duration of anaesthesia. The risk of toxicity is usually less due to rapid clearance from the circulation. It can be safely used when large volumes are needed or in intravenous regional anaesthesia. The safe maximum dose is 7 mg/kg and 8.5 mg/kg with adrenaline, (400 mg and 600 mg respectively).

Various solutions are available for injection in different strengths ranging from 0.5 to 2%. Even 3 or 4% solutions are used for dental anaesthesia. The addition of vasoconstrictor may increase its duration of action significantly. It is also a constituent of EMLA cream (a mixture, of equal amounts of crystalline 2.5% prilocaine and 2.5% lignocaine).

Doses in excess of 600 mg may cause methaemoglobinaemia due to its metabolite orthotoluidine. This can be rapidly reversed by IV administration of methylene blue 1 mg/kg.

Prilocaine should not be used for epidural block in obstetrics because of the need for repeat dosing.

## Bupivacaine

Bupivacaine is a new amide local anaesthetic with a slow onset and a long duration of action, about 3 hours. It has increased lipid solubility and protein binding activity compared to lignocaine. It tends to produce more sensory block than motor block. It is highly potent.

It is available as 0.25%, 0.5% and 0.75% solution. It is mainly used in infiltration anaesthesia, peripheral nerve block, spinal and epidural block. It is not recommended for use in intravenous regional anaesthesia. The safe maximum dose is 2 mg/kg for single injection and 2.5 mg/kg with the addition of adrenaline. The addition of adrenaline has only a marginal effect. Epidural bupivacaine is widely used for obstetric analgesia, but 0.75% strength is not recommended as the safe maximum total dose is easily exceeded. It has low placental transfer.

Bupivacaine may be associated with frequent cardiotoxic reactions particularly when the safe maximum dose is exceeded.

## Mepivacaine

It is a good local anaesthetic. The onset of action is usually rapid and duration of effect may range from 2 to 3 hours. It is less toxic than lignocaine. It produces vasoconstriction to some extent and thus addition of vasoconstrictor is not needed.

It can be used in various types of block.
(a) in filtration anaesthesia 0.5 to 1%
(b) nerve block 2 to 3%
(c) spinal block 4% (heavy)
(d) caudal and epidural block 1.5 to 2%

Maximum safe dose is 400 mg, about 5 mg/kg. It is not effective in topical use. Side effects are usually mild. It may pass through placental barrier. It should not be used in obstetric analgesia. The drug is not much used nowadays.

## Etidocaine

It is a new potent amide local anaesthetic with a rapid onset and long duration of action, about 2 to 4 hours. It is highly protein bound and has high oil/water partition coefficient. The depth and duration of motor blockade exceeds those of sensory block. Thus, it is helpful in operations where muscle relaxation is much needed. It is mostly used in infiltration, nerve block, and epidural anaesthesia.

The maximum single dose for infiltration is 300 mg in adults. It is not used for topical anaesthesia and spinal anaesthesia.

## Ropivacaine

It is also a new potent amide local anaesthetic structurally similar to mepivacaine and bupivacaine. Its pKa and plasma protein binding are almost similar to those of bupivacaine. It is less lipid soluble. Its onset of action is slow and duration of effect is long, about 4 to 8 hours.

It can be used in infiltration, peripheral nerve block, spinal and epidural anaesthesia. It may cause local vasoconstriction. The safe dose is 150 to 200 mg. It is available in solutions of 0.5 to 2%. No serious cardiovascular adverse effects are found. It is eliminated more rapidly than bupivacaine.

## Cocaine

Cocaine is not used for regional anaesthesia due to its toxicity and addiction. It is an ester and is used as topical anaesthesia. It causes intense vasoconstriction. It is used in surface ENT procedures and for anaesthetising nasal mucosa before nasotracheal intubation.

It is used solely as a surface anaesthetic (4%). Its maximum dose is 100 mg. The addition of adrenaline is not recommended.

## Procaine

It is an ester local anaesthetic of rapid onset and short to medium duration of action. It is not used nowadays. It is poorly absorbed from the mucous membrane and is not used topically. It is rapidly hydrolysed by plasma pseudocholinesterase. It can be used safely in large quantity without systemic toxicity. It provides vasodilation and antiarrhythmic activity.

## Chloroprocaine

It is an ester local anaesthetic of rapid onset and short duration of action. It is relative less toxic due to plasma hydrolysis. It can be used for short lasting infiltration anaesthesia and nerve blocks. It is not recommended for spinal anaesthesia as it can damage nerve roots and cause permanent paraplegia. Maximum dose is 800 mg, increasing to 1000 mg with adrenaline.

## Amethocaine (Tetracaine)

It is also a potent long acting local anaesthetic. It can be used for spinal anaesthesia in isobaric, hypobaric and hyperbaric solutions. It provides rapid onset, good sensory anaesthesia and profound muscular paralysis. Duration of action ranges from 2 to 4 hours. Addition of adrenaline can extend the duration to 4 to 6 hours.

It is also a useful agent for topical anaesthesia. It can be used for corneal and endotracheal topical anaesthesia.

It is rapidly absorbed from vascular mucous membranes and cause systemic toxicity. With the introduction of bupivacaine, the drug is rarely used nowadays.

# CHAPTER 3

# Equipment for Regional Anaesthesia

## INTRODUCTION

Regional anaesthesia may sometimes be hazardous due to failure of block, inadequate anaesthesia and may be complicated with cardiovascular and neurological toxicity. Sudden cardiovascular collapse and anaphylactic shock can occur. General anaesthesia may be instituted in cases with failure or inadequate block. Thus, the following equipment should be available.

1. Equipment for general anaesthesia.
   - (a) Anaesthesia machine
   - (b) Laryngoscopes
   - (c) Set of endotracheal tubes
   - (d) Endotracheal connections
   - (e) Catheter mount
   - (f) Suction apparatus
   - (g) Gas cylinders, $O_2$ cylinder
2. Monitoring equipment, ECG machine, pulse oximeters, blood pressure monitors.
3. Cardiorespiratory resuscitation equipment
4. Defibrillator, pacemaker
5. Intravenous drugs, muscle relaxants
6. *Emergency drugs*: vasopressors, adrenaline, steroids. IV infusion fluid
7. IV infusion set, IV catheters

The description of all these are not within the scope of this presentation. Anaesthetists seem to be well-oriented with such equipment and drugs.

## EQUIPMENT FOR REGIONAL ANAESTHESIA

1. Nerve block needles
2. Nerve stimulator for nerve blocks

3. Spinal needle
4. Epidural needle, Tuohy needle
5. Epidural catheter, filter, syringe
6. Patient controlled analgesia.

## NERVE BLOCK NEEDLES

These are special needles used in regional anaesthesia to identify a nerve plexus or peripheral nerve. These are made of steel with luer-lock arrangement. These are small in diameter 22 gauze or less and long enough (50 mm or 120 mm) to reach the intended nerve or plexus.

They have short and somewhat blunt bevels as it causes less trauma to nerve tissue. Short bevel 45° nerve (Fig. 3.1) block needle (22G) is preferred. These have translucent hubs as it aids early detection of intravascular injection. A side port may be there for injection of the local anaesthetic.

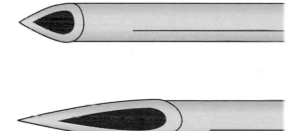

**Fig. 3.1:** Bevel of nerve block needle.
Blunt bevel on top preferred

A security bead on the needle shaft may be there to prevent retraction of a distal needle segment below the skin, if it breaks at the hub.

Needles include an attachment for the electrode of nerve stimulator which aids in localising the nerve. It may be Teflon coated insulated with an exposed tip. Noninsulated needles are also available in wide variety of length and diameter. These are being used satisfactorily, but for deep nerves it is better to use insulated needles. Insulated needles are usually with greater diameter and thus these are liable to cause more nerve injury. In cases of noninsulated needle the current passes through the shaft along with its tip. When a nerve is stimulated through the shaft, the local anaesthetic solution may be placed well away from the nerve and thus may cause unsuccessful block.

## Procedure

The nerve block needle is gently passed through the skin and subcutaneous tissue. The lead of the nerve stimulator is attached and initial output is selected from it. The needle is advanced gently towards nerve to get the nerve stimulation. The output is adjusted to get the maximum stimulation with minimum output. The blunt needle point is fixed and the local anaesthetic solution is injected. Nerve stimulation may be reduced to some extent due to displacement of the nerve from the tip of needle.

Catheters can be introduced and placed in desired space after proper localising the nerve. Continuous infusion of local anaesthetic may be helpful in some cases.

Paraesthesia may be there due to contact of nerve with the needle tip when nerve stimulator is not used. It is better to avoid to elicit paraesthesia as it increases the risk of nerve injury.

- *Immobile needle technique:* Here one anaesthetist helps to maintain the needle in position and the other injects the local anaesthetic solution through the side port. It reduces the risk of misplacement and intravascular injection. It is used mostly for major nerve blocks in deeper planes where large amount of solutions are to be deposited.

## SYRINGES

Syringes with finger rings are mostly helpful as these allow single handed loading and performing repeated aspiration tests, while the other hand may be used to stabilise the needle. Standard syringes need some assistance to aspirate and inject along with the use of flexible extension tubing to prevent the movement of the needle tip during the procedure.

- Simple infiltration of local anaesthetic solution around bony, vascular or fascial landmarks where precise location of nerves are not certain, can be done by using standard needles used for intramuscular injections and standard syringes.

## PERIPHERAL NERVE STIMULATOR FOR NERVE BLOCKS (LONGNECKER & MURPHY, 1997) (FIG. 3.2)

The equipment is meant to produce a visible muscular contraction at a low power electrical stimuli to locate the nerve plexus or peripheral nerve.

1. It is designed safe, practical and portable for routine clinical use.
2. It is battery-powered.
3. It provides two leads, one to the skin and the other to the locating needle (cathode –ve). The polarity of the

leads should be clearly indicated and color coded. The leads can be detached and sterilised.

4. It can be used in wide variety of needles.
5. It provides digital display of delivered current and/or voltage with linear output below 1 mA.
6. Voltage 9 V and current 5 mA limited to cope with different body tissue resistances. A small current of 0.5 mA or less is used with a frequency of 1 to 2 Hz.
7. Short duration impulse less than 100 μsec at frequency of 1 to 2 Hz to stimulate motor nerves preferentially to sensory nerves.

*Note:*
• Usually a small current (0.25 to 0.5 mA) is used to stimulate the motor nerves. The frequency is set at 1 to 2 Hz. Tetanic stimuli are not used to avoid discomfort. The duration of stimulus is short 1 to 2 ms for painless motor contraction.
• The location of nerve can be accurately judged while using low currents. Success rate, even in technically difficult nerve blocks is mostly satisfactory.

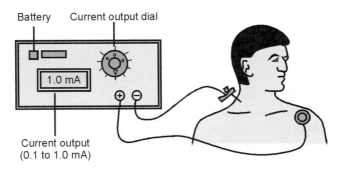

**Fig. 3.2:** Nerve stimulator

## Common Uses of Nerve Stimulator for Nerve Blocks

1. Brachial plexus block
2. Suprascapular nerve block
3. Sciatic nerve block
4. Femoral nerve block
5. Popliteal fossa block
6. Obutator nerve block
7. Radial nerve block
8. Median nerve block
9. Trigeminal nerve block, etc.

- Nerve stimulator used for monitoring of neuromuscular block can be used provided it can provide 0.1 to 3 mA with a display of the current. It should to noted that high output stimulators can damage the nerve tissue.

- Higher current, if used can stimulate the nerve fibres even when needletip is well away from the nerve. Muscle fibres can also be stimulated. All these will lead to failure of block.

- Anaesthetist should have a sound knowledge and skill regarding the subject to perform regional anaesthesia using nerve stimulator. He should know which muscles are to contract from the stimulation of the target nerve.

## Procedure

The negative lead from the stimulator is attached to the insulated block needle and the other lead (anode +ve) is attached to the patient well away from the site of needle insertion. It will ensure that the current flows through the path of the nerve.

Battery power is tested and circuit integrity is checked. The delivered current is set at a moderate level (3 mA or less).

As the needletip approaches the nerve, the electric current induces stimulation producing muscle contraction. While using low current 3 mA or less the nerve will not be stimulated, if the needle tip is more than 1 cm distant. Pulse synchronous movement with low power levels indicate the position of the needle tip close to the nerve. The minimum stimulating current and voltage may vary with the type of nerves (superficial or deep).

When the nerve is located accurately, the needle is stabilised and aspiration test is done. Then the local anaesthetic solution is injected gently. There may be initial increased muscle movement as the local anaesthetic increases the conductivity. Thereafter, there is quick fade of muscle movements due to displaced nerve by the injection and increased nerve needle distance.

- Pain and resistance to flow may indicate inaccurate needle position. The location of the needle should be readjusted.
- Nerve blocks may be done even when the patient is sedated or anaesthetised as the response is visibly monitored. There is no need to elicit pain or paraesthesia. Extreme care is needed to avoid neural damage. Needle tip should be adjusted close to the nerve but not to touch the nerve.

## SPINAL NEEDLE (FIG. 3.3)

This needle is used to inject local anaesthetic solution into the subarachnoid space. Opioids can also be injected through it. Lumbar puncture is also indicated to sample CSF, to administer antibiotics and cytotoxic intrathecally. It is also used for therapeutic purposes to reduce the intracranial pressure.

**Fig. 3.3:** Spinal needle

It is a long needle (7.5 to 10 cm) with a narrow bore (22 to 25 SWG) and carries a fine wire stylet upto the bevel of needle. It includes a transparent hub to detect the flow of CSF quickly. The stylet is used to prevent tissue occluding during introduction. It also strengthens the needle shaft. The stylet is withdrawn when needletip is in the subarachnoid space. Paediatric variety of 5 cm length is also available. Extra large of 15 cm is used for obese patients.

These needles are available in different sizes from 18 G to 29G in diameter. The needles of 25 G or smaller should be used with introducer which is usually 18-19 G. The 22 G or 25 G needles are commonly used. The 22 G needle is little rigid and easy to direct. It gives a better feel while passing through different tissues. The CSF is slower to pass through smaller sized needles.

The bevel may be either cutting traumatic or non-cutting atraumatic pencil point with a side hole (injection port) just proximal to tip. The pencil point needle have a tapered tip and requires more force to introduce. It may be difficult to differentiate the structures. These needles cause less damage to the dura and thus lower the risk of postspinal headache. These needles are specially indicated in headache prone patients, aged patients, obstetric cases and in outpatient clinics. Traumatic bevel needles cut the durameter causing a ragged tear which may allow CSF leakage and cause postspinal headache. Atraumatic needle usually separates rather than cut the longitudinal dural fibres and the gap usually seals following the removal of needles.

Selection of appropriate needle gauze is also important to reduce the incidence of post-spinal headache. 25 G needle seems to be more beneficial in this respect.

* A prepacked sterile disposable kit for spinal anaesthesia may be readily available. It should contain:
  1. One galley pot to keep antiseptic lotions
  2. Towels, towel clips, sponge holding forceps, swab cotton, gauge. These are for antiseptic cleaning and draping
  3. Syringes with hypodermic needles
  4. Ampoules or vials of local anaesthetic drug
  5. Spinal needle/Tuohy needle
  6. Some drug vials: adrenaline, bupivacaine, lignocaine, etc.

All spinal needles should be tested for temper before sterilisation. While sterilising particularly by boiling, stylet should be in place since this will protect the needle point.

## EPIDURAL NEEDLES (FIG. 3.4)

These needles are used to identify and cannulate the epidural space. The Tuohy variety is being widely used for epidural block. It is also meant for administration of opioids in epidural space.

The needle is 10 cm in length with a shaft of 8 cm with 1 cm markings. A 15 cm variety is also available for use in obese patients. Here the needle wall is thin to allow cannulation through it. It also provides a stylet introducer.

The bevel is made slightly oblique at 20° to the shaft with a rather blunt leading edge. Usually 16G or 18G needles are popularly used.

**Fig. 3.4:** Tuohy epidural needle

The markings help to determine the distance between skin and epidural space. Thus, the length of catheter left in epidural space can be roughly judged. The particular shape of the bevel aids to direct the catheter easily in the epidural space. The blunt tip minimises the risk of inadvertent dural puncture. A paediatric variety 19 G, 5 cm long, Tuohy needle is available with 0.5 cm markings. It allows the passage of a 21G nylon catheter.

- **Caution**: If withdrawal of catheter is needed through the needle, the needle should be withdrawn along with the catheter, otherwise there is risk of transection of catheter by the oblique bevel.

## EPIDURAL CATHETER (FIG. 3.5)

It is a transparent malleable nylon/Teflon tube. It is 90 cm in length. It should be biologically inert and cause no adverse reactions and safe to use. The tip is closed and rounded and there are two side ports at the distal end. The distal end of the catheter is marked at 5 cm intervals with 1 cm divisions between 5 to 15 cm. The proximal end of epidural catheter may be attached to a luer lock syringe and a filter.

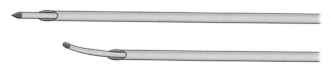

**Fig. 3.5:** Catheter inside the spinal needles

Epidural catheter with or without a stylet is passed 2 to 4 cm into the epidural space. The epidural needle should be removed over the catheter. The catheter should never be withdrawn through the epidural needle as it may shear off and remain within the epidural space. After withdrawal, the catheter should be inspected for any signs of breakage.

### Caution

1. The catheter should match appropriate gauze of needles.
2. Markings help the desired length of catheter within the epidural space, usually 2 to 4 cm.
3. Catheter with sharp point with single port at distant point may increase the risk of dural or vascular puncture.
4. Catheters should be tested for patency before use.
5. Catheter can puncture the dura.
6. Both needle and catheter should be withdrawn at one time at the time of need.
7. Direction of epidural catheter within the epidural space cannot be predicted.
8. The catheter should not be advanced for more than 5 cm within the epidural space.

## EPIDURAL FILTER AND SYRINGE

The proximal end of the epidural catheter should be connected with a filter. This is usually a 0.22 micron mesh bacterial, viral and foreign bodies filter. If used for long periods, it should be changed every 24 hours to ensure better safety.

The syringe is used for the purpose of easy identification of epidural space by loss of resistance test using either air or saline. This should be low resistance plunger syringe. Plastic or glass syringes are available. These must be properly sterilised before use.

## PATIENT CONTROLLED ANALGESIA

Patient controlled analgesia is the most recent advancement in the management of postoperative pain and chronic pain syndromes. It allows the patient to control drug delivery according to his own requirements. A PCA machine can administer a preset dose of drug when he presses the button. The machine incorporates a microprocessor which prevents misuse or overdose. PCA provides satisfactory analgesia with minimum side effects. It can be used for IM, subcutaneous, IV and epidural administration. It operates on mains or battery. Alarms are included for malfunction, obstruction and disconnection. The PCA is programmed by the experienced anaesthetist.

The machine essentially includes a pump with an accuracy of at least ±5% of the programmed dose, the remote demand button connected to the pump and activated by the patient. It should have an antisiphon and back flow valve. It should have memory capabilities. Tamper resistant features are also included. To prevent overdosage, dose and lockout controls are activated only with the use of a key or by placing a numerical combination into the machine.

The administration of analgesic may be either patient controlled bolus administration on demand or continuous basal infusion and patient controlled bolus administration.

### Caution

1. The PCA machine should be accurate and reliable. All safety measures should be included.

2. It should operate on mains/battery.
3. Technical errors may be fatal.
4. Patient should co-operate and understand the procedure sincerely.
5. Patient should be able to administer the drug as required. He should be properly trained to use the machine. It should be noted that complete pain-free condition may not be achieved in chronic pain syndrome cases but tolerability of pain should be kept within safe limits.
6. Although the patient is medicating himself, the anaesthetist should retain control over doses and lock-out intervals.

# CHAPTER 4

# Spinal Anaesthesia

## DEFINITION

Spinal anaesthesia may be defined as that regional anaesthesia obtained by blocking the spinal nerves in the subarachnoid space. Local anaesthetic is deposited in subarachnoid space to act on the spinal nerve roots.

## ANATOMICAL CONSIDERATIONS OF SPINE

### Vertebral Column  (Fig. 4.1)

The vertebral column consists of 33 bones, seven cervical, twelve thoracic, five lumbar, five sacral and four coccygeal vertebrae. Five are fused to form sacrum and four to form coccyx. The sacrum and coccyx are said to be the distal extensions of the vertebral column.

### *Vertebra*

A *vertebra* consists of a body and an arch that comprises two pedicles anteriorly and two laminae posteriorly. Transverse processes arise from the junction of pedicles and laminae. Spinous process arises from the point of union of the laminae in the posterior midline. The laminae and spinous processes are joined by ligament. But the pedicles form gaps (intervertebral foramina) through which the spinal nerves exit the spinal canal. In the lumbar region the spinous processes are mostly horizontal. So the needle should be introduced at this region and directed at right angles to the sagittal plane.

### *Intervertebral Fibrocartilages*

*Intervertebral fibrocartilages* (discs) are interposed between adjacent surfaces of the vertebral bodies. The vertebral column

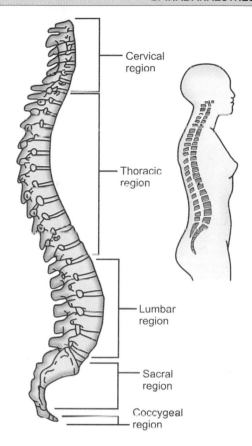

**Fig. 4.1:** Vertebral column

is lengthened by these discs. These may comprise one-third to a quarter of its total length and give the vertebral column its flexibility. The shape of column largely dependent on these discs.

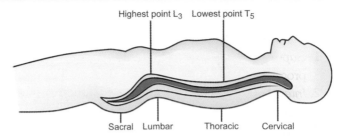

Highest point $L_3$    Lowest point $T_5$

Sacral    Lumbar        Thoracic    Cervical

**Fig. 4.2:** Curves of vertebral canal

Vertebral column has 4 curves (Fig. 4.2). Thoracic and sacral curves are primary and exist at birth. These are concave anteriorly. Cervical and lumbar curves are secondary, develop after birth. These are convex anteriorly. When the patient is lying supine and horizontal, the high point of the spinal curve is at the level of $L_3$ and the low point is at $T_5$. The degree of curvature may vary in different individuals and can be modified by posture. In fully flexed spine, the cervical and lumbar curves are obliterated. Pregnant women have an exaggerated lumbar curve. In old age discs atrophy and this may give rise to bowed back of old age. Abnormal curves may include kyphosis, lordosis or scoliosis and these may cause difficulty in lumbar puncture.

### *Vertebral Canal*

Vertebral canal is bounded anteriorly by vertebral bodies and discs, posteriorly by arch bearing spinous processes and interspinous ligament and laterally by pedicles and laminae. It contains:

1. Spinal nerve roots
2. Spinal cord with enclosing membranes.
3. Blood vessels, fat, areolar tissue in extradural space.

## *Vertebral Ligaments*

Vertebral ligaments bounding the vertebral canal are as follows:

1. *Supraspinous ligament:* They connect the tips of spinous processes.
2. *Interspinous ligament:* It connects the posterior spinous processes.
4. *Ligamentum flavum:* It connects the laminae of the vertebrae. They become progressively thicker from above downwards.
5. Posterior longitudinal ligament: It is within the vertebral canal on the posterior surface of vertebral bodies.
6. Anterior longitudinal ligament: It runs in front of the vertebral bodies and intervertebral discs.

- During midline insertion of a needle into the subarachnoid space the following structures are traversed:
  1. Skin
  2. Subcutaneous tissue
  3. Supraspinous ligament
  4. Interspinous ligament
  5. Ligamentum flavum
  6. Areolar tissue of epidural space
  7. Dura mater of spinal cord

In lateral approach supraspinous ligament and interspinous ligament are not encountered.

## Spinal Cord

It is the elongated part of the central nervous system, an ovoid column of nervous tissue about 45 cm long, flattened anteroposteriorly extending from the medulla at foramen magnum up to the second lumbar vertebra in the spinal canal.

It ends in conus medullaries from which filum terminale descends down to coccyx. *Cauda equina* is the terminal part of spinal cord along with lower lumbar and sacral nerve roots within the spinal canal (Fig. 4.3).

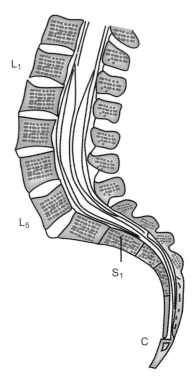

**Fig. 4.3:** Lower part of vertebral canal and spinal cord

Lumbar puncture above $L_2$ and $L_3$ interspace should be avoided as it may cause cord injury. The spinal cord is enclosed three membrane from outside inwards, dura mater, arachnoid mater and pia mater.

Spinal dura mater is the continuation downward of the inner meningeal layer of cranial dura mater. Above it is attached to the margins of foramen magnum and below it ends at the level of $S_2$. It is separated from the bony wall of vertebral column by the *extradural space*. Actually it is formed by splitting of two layers of dura. It contains fat, areolar tissue, a venous plexus and anterior and posterior roots of spinal nerves. Dura is mainly composed of longitudinal fibres so the spinal needle should be introduced with the bevel to separate the fibres rather than be dividing the fibres.

*Arachnoid mater* is thin, delicate, nonvascular and transparent membrane closely adherent to dura mater. The space (subdural) is usually a capillary layer.

*Pia mater* is the innermost layer closely adherent to the spinal cord. Pia mater is separated from arachnoid mater by the subarachnoid space. Pia mater ends as filum terminale which pierces the distal end of dural sac and is attached to coccyx.

The *subarachnoid space* is annular in the cervical and thoracic region and about 3 mm deep, below the first lumbar the space is circular. Local anaesthetic solution is deposited here in spinal analgesia. The space is filled with cerebrospinal fluid and traversed by cobweb trabeculae, denticulate ligaments and by spinal nerve roots. It communicates with the ventricular system of brain by foramen of Magendie, foramen of Lushka and foramina of Key and Retzius.

The spinal cord consists 31 pairs spinal segments according to spinal nerves which arise from it. The nerve roots within the dura mater have no epineural sheaths.

(a) Cervical–8 pairs

(b) Thoracic–12 pairs

(c) Lumbar–5 pairs

(d) Sacral–5 pairs

(e) Coccygeal–1 pair

## Spinal Nerves (Fig. 4.4)

There are 31 pairs of spinal nerves each arising from the cord by anterior and porterior roots. Each spinal nerve supplies a specific skin area or dermatome and skeletal muscles.

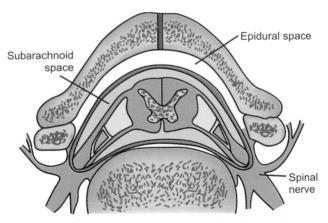

**Fig. 4.4:** Subarachnoid and epidural space

Anterior spinal root is efferent containing:

(a) Motor to voluntary muscles.

(b) Preganglionic sympathetic fibres ($T_1$ to $L_2$ or $L_3$) travel with spinal nerves before leaving to form the sympathetic chain. The sympathetic chain extends the whole length of spinal cord along the anterolateral side of the vertebral bodies. It gives rise to stellate ganglion, splanchnic nerves and coeliac plexus.

## *Posterior Spinal Root*

All the afferent impulses from the entire body including viscera pass into the posterior roots. Each porterior root has a ganglion.

The anterior and posterior roots join in the intervertebral foramina to form spinal nerve trunks. They divide into anterior and porterior divisions of mixed nerves.

The dermatome of the body signifies a segmental skin area innervated by various spinal cord segments. Segmental levels of some important regions are as follows:

1. Clavicle $C_3$
2. Second intercostal space $T_2$
3. Nipple line $T_4$ $T_5$
4. Subcostal arch $T_7$ $T_8$
5. Umbilicus $T_{10}$
6. Inguinal region $L_1$
7. Perineum $S_{1-4}$

## The Epidural Space

It is formed by the splitting of the two layers of the spinal dura. The space is limited above by the fusion of two layers of dura at foramen magnum and below by the sacrococcygeal ligament closing the sacral hiatus. It contains:

1. 31 pairs of spinal nerve roots with their dural prolongations.
2. Venous plexuses of the vertebral canal.
3. Areolar and fatty tissues between arteries, veins and nerves. Greatest depth of fatty tissue in epidural space lies posteriorly and anterolaterally. It is continuous with the fat around the spinal nerves in the intervertebral foramina.

The negative intrathoracic pressure is transmitted through the paravertebral spaces to the thoracic epidural space. It is diminished to some extent in cervical and lumbar regions. The presence of negative pressure in epidural space often aids to detect the space during administration of epidural injections.

## Cerebrospinal Fluid

It is derived from the choroid plexuses of the third, fourth and lateral ventricles either by secretion, filtration or dialysation. A small amount may be obtained from perivascular spaces.

The fluid is passed into the venous sinuses by arachnoid villi, granulation and mesothetial cells. It is also removed into lymph stream through the pacchionian bodies.

- Circulation of cerebrospinal fluid: The fluid formed by choroid plexuses in lateral ventricles passes through foramen of Monro. It mixes with the fluid formed in third ventricle. Thereafter it passes through aqueduct of Sylvius to the fourth ventricle. Then it reaches the subarachnoid space through the central foramen of Magendie and the lateral foramina of Lushka, key and Retzius to reach the cisterna magna. It circulates the whole brain and is absorbed in venous sinuses through the arachnoidal villi. It should be noted that this circulation does not affect the spinal analgesia in any way.

### *Physical Properties of CSF*

1. Clear, colourless fluid
2. Specific grasity 1003–1009
3. Quantity 120 to 150 in adult
   (a) volume of spinal CSF about 25 ml to 30 ml
   (b) volume in ventricles 60 to 75 ml
   (c) volume in large cisternal reservoirs 35 to 45 ml
4. Average pressure 100 to 150 mm water

5. *Alkaline:* pH 7.6
6. *Chemical:*
   Protein 24–40 mg/100 ml
   Sugar 45–80 mg%
   Sodium Chloride 750 mg%
   Urea 10–30 mg%
   Bicarbonate 24 mEq/L
7. Drugs are not secreted into it.
8. Bile is not found in it even in deep jaundice
9. Antibiotics are not found in CSF.

### Functions of CSF

1. Acts as fluid cushion to protect the brain.
2. Regulates the volume of cranial contents.
3. May have little effect in metabolic exchanges of nervous tissue.

## INDICATIONS OF SPINAL ANAESTHESIA

1. *Location and nature of surgery:* It is particularly helpful in abdominal surgery and surgery of pelvis, perineum and lower extremities as it provides excellent muscular relaxation. Surgery of upper abdomen, chest, shoulder and upper extremities can be done, but with some difficulty as it may interfere with respiration and circulation.
2. *Patient's choice attitude:* Patients cooperation is highly desired. Anxious apprehensive patients or patients with psychological disorders are bad choice for spinal anaesthesia.

3. *Age of the patient:* Adults patients are good subjects and geriatric patients may be benefitted with spinal/epidural block. Children may need light general anaesthesia along with regional anaesthesia.

4. *Medical disorders*: Patients with heart, lung, liver and kidney diseases tolerate spinal anaesthesia better in comparison to general anaesthesia. However, the relative merits and demerits are to be wisely balanced.

5. *Pain evaluation with differential spinal block*

6. *Therapeutic management in patients with chronic pain syndromes.*

## CONTRAINDICATIONS OF SPINAL ANAESTHESIA

1. Patients with marked disorders of central nervous system such as brain tumour, meningitis, etc. Patients with increased intracranial pressure may have a risk of brain stem herniation.

2. Infected skin condition in lumbar region.

3. Septicaemia, bacteremia.

4. Patients with documented allergy with local anaesthetics.

5. Patients with shock, hypovolaemia.

6. Patients with clotting abnormalities.

7. Preexisting neurologic diseases.

8. Inability to obtain valid consent for spinal anaesthesia is the absolute contraindication.

## PHYSIOLOGICAL EFFECTS OF SPINAL ANALGESIA

1. Spinal anaesthesia blocks sensory, motor and sympathetic nerve fibres. The small diameter nonmyelinated fibres (sympathetic) are more sensitive than larger myelinated (sensory and motor) fibres. Sympathetic block usually exceeds somatic sensory by two or more dermatomes. Weaker concentration of local anaesthetic may block sensation without providing motor paralysis. With the sufficient increase in dose and concentration, both anterior and porterior nerve roots are blocked with intense anaesthesia (sensory) and motor paralysis.

   Differences in levels of block for the different nerve modalities can occur following spinal anaesthesia. Preganglionic sympathetic block is usually more diffuse and may extend 2 to 4 segments above the block. It is usually first in onset and last to abolish. Motor nerve block is mostly 1 to 4 segments below the sensory levels.

   Sequence of different nerve fibre block is usually in the following order:

   (a) Vasomotor block
   (b) Pain
   (c) Tactile
   (d) Motor
   (e) Pressure
   (f) Proprioception

2. Vasomotor paralysis is proportional to the degree of sympathetic paralysis.

3. A reduction of blood loss is most common in case of spinal anaesthesia. It is mostly due to sympathetic nervous

system block which causes decreased venous return to the heart and decreased cardiac output. Decreased systemic vascular resistance and bradycardia are also the other factors.

4. Resting alveolar ventilation is mostly unchanged, but in high spinal block abdominal and intercostal muscles are paralysed leading to decreased ability to cough and expel the secretions. The patient may complain of difficulty in breathing.

5. Spinal anaesthesia above the level of $T_5$ inhibits sympathetic nerves of gastrointestinal tract. Unopposed parasympathetic activity causes contraction of intestine and released sphincters. Ureters are contracted and ureterovesical sphincters are relaxed.

6. Adrenocortical response to surgery is absent due to block of afferent impulses in spinal anaesthesia.

7. There is overall reduction of bleeding at the site of operation due to decreased blood pressure.

8. Increased blood flow to lower extremities following sympathetic nervous system block is observed.

9. In low spinal anaesthesia, bladder and urogenital dysfunction may result due to lower thoracolumbar sympathetic and sacral parasympathetic inactivation.

## ADVANTAGES OF SPINAL ANAESTHESIA OVER GENERAL ANAESTHESIA

1. Spinal anaesthesia permits the patient to remain awake during surgery.

2. Spinal analgesia is technically easy to perform and provides reliable and rapid anaesthesia.

3. Spinal anaesthesia reduces the risk of aspiration. Pulmonary complications are always less.

4. Various systemic medications are needed in general anaesthesia, but in spinal block it is usually significantly less.

5. Patients with metabolic disorders tolerate spinal anaesthesia better.

6. The metabolic response to surgery is not significant in spinal anaesthesia.

7. Decreased blood levels of glucose, insulin, free fatty acid and cortisol are evident in spinal anaesthesia.

8. Decreased blood level of adrenaline and noradrenaline is found in upper thoracic spinal block, but no change in lower thoracic block.

9. Blood loss is usually less in spinal anaesthesia.

10. Requirement of blood transfusion is less in spinal block. Thus, associated complications are also less.

11. Incidence of postoperative thromboembolic complications is less in spinal block.

12. Mortality rate seems to be less in spinal anaesthesia.

## COMPLICATIONS OF SPINAL ANAESTHESIA

Complications associated with spinal anaesthesia are well recognised and these are as follows:

1. Hypotension
2. Postspinal headache
3. High spinal
4. Nausea/vomiting
5. Backache
6. Urinary retention

## Comparison between spinal anaesthesia and epidural anaesthesia

| | Spinal | Epidural |
|---|---|---|
| 1. Technic | Easy Fine needle can be used. Reliable | Relatively difficult Larger gauge needle needed. Identification of epidural space needs extra skill. |
| 2. Local anaesthetic | Less volume | Large volume Toxicity significant |
| 3. Degree of block | Toxicity less Intense, complete | Less intense, rarely complete |
| 4. Onset of block | Fast (2-8 min) | Slow (20-30 min) |
| 5. Duration of action | Variable depends on agent used. But prolonged using catheters. | Prolonged using catheters |
| 6. Quality of block | Satisfoctory No segmental block | Patchy block common Muscle relaxation is not complete. |
| 7. Headache | Postspinal head-ache common | Less common |
| 8. Neurologic sequalae | Less | Less |
| 9. Spread of block | Predictable | Less predictable |
| 10. Urinary retention | Frequent | Less frequent |
| 11. Hypotension | More profound | Less |
| 12. Failure rate | Less/nil | Greater mostly due to technical problems |
| 13. Backache | Frequent | Less frequent |

7. Neurologic sequelae: haematoma, abscess, septic meningitis, aseptic meningitis, neurotrauma, spinal cord ischaemia.
8. Hypoventilation
9. Paraesthesia
10. Failure/inadequate analgesia.

## Hypotension

It is the most common complication of spinal anaesthesia. It is mostly due to sympathetic nervous system block ($T_1$ to $L_2$) that diminishes venous return to heart and decreases cardiac output or decreases systemic vascular resistance. *Bradycardia* due to block of cardioaccelerator sympathetic nerve fibres and decreased venous return to heart may be the added factor to produce decreased cardiac output and hypotension. The degree of hypotension increases with the extent of spinal block. Hypovolaemia, head up tilt, high spinal analgesia, certain drugs like opioids etc. enhance hypotensive effect. A saddle block should not produce hypotension.

Early treatment is essential and it should include the following:

1. Head up posture should be corrected.
2. IV fluids
3. Pressor agents
4. Alpha and beta adrenergic agonists: ephedrine
5. Atropine to treat bradycardia
6. Phenylephrine (an $\alpha$ adrenergic agonist) may also be used.

## Postspinal Headache

It usually occurs 2 to 7 days after lumbar puncture and may persist for up to 6 weeks. It is frontal or occipital or global and worse in sitting and standing posture. It may be associated with diplopia, vertigo, tinnitus, photophobia and impaired hearing. Postspinal headache is mostly due to decreased intracranial tension caused by leakage of CSF through the dural hole created by lumbar puncture. Diplopia is due to traction of abducens nerve.

The incidence of postspinal headache is always low following use of 25 gauze needles in spinal puncture.

### Management

1. Bed rest. Supine position improves pain. Sitting or standing position exacerbates pain
2. Large fluid intake oral of IV
3. Analgesics
4. Use of extradural infusion of sterile saline
5. Extradural blood patch
6. Administration of caffeine sodium benzoate (500 mg IV) may alleviate headache in most cases.

## High Spinal

It is due to excessive cephalad spread of local anaesthetic in the CSF. Unrecognised dural puncture during epidural anaesthesia or migration of epidural catheter into subarachnoid space may be the other causes.

Clinical features develop very rapidly particularly when large volume of local anaesthetic is injected rapidly. Manifestations include hypotension, difficulty in breathing, apnoea, nausea/vomiting, unconsciousness and even cardiac arrest.

- Prevention should be tried with the following:
  1. Use of correct dose, strength and volume of local anaesthetic solution.
  2. Placement of catheter in correct site.
  3. Careful monitoring of vital signs is essential and early detection is needed to tackle the case.

*Management*

1. Positive pressure ventilation
2. Adequate oxygenation
3. IV fluids, head down tilt
4. Administer pressor drugs
5. Treat bradycardia
6. Immediate CPR in cases of cardiac arrest.

## Nausea/Vomiting

Nausea and vomiting may occur in the early period following spinal anaesthesia.

Cerebral ischaemia due to hypotension may be responsible. It is usually treated with IV fluids and administration of sympathomimetics.

Predominant parasympathetic activity as a result of selective sympathetic block in gastrointestinal tract may produce nausea/vomiting. Atropine may be extremely helpful in such cases.

Local anaesthetic solution when combined with vaso-constrictors may increase the incidence of nausea and vomiting.

## Backache

It occurs frequently following spinal anaesthesia. It is only mild or moderate intensity and does not last long. It may be related to ligament strain due to positioning needed for surgery. Muscle spasm and muscle haematoma may be the other factors. Severe back pain needs immediate neurological investigations.

### Urinary Retention

This may occur following spinal anaesthesia as it interferes the innervation of urinary bladder and urethral sphincter particularly when sensory and motor block recovers before bladder function. Administration of large volumes of IV fluid aggravates bladder distension. Use of a bladder catheter usually prevents this uncomfortable condition.

### Paraesthesia

It may occur due to touching the nerve with the injection needle or during injection of the anaesthetic solution. There is intense pain and shock suggesting that the needle may be against nerve root. In that case the needle point should be removed and placed in another suitable interspace, otherwise there may be injury and permanent nerve damage.

### Hypoventilation

Ventilatory impairment may be due to hypotension leading to impaired medullary blood flow and hypoxia of the respiratory centre. Phrenic nerve block, intercostal and diaphragmatic paralysis may also occur in high spinal anaesthesia. In such cases constant monitoring is essential for early detection. Positive pressure ventilation and adequate oxygenation may be needed in these cases.

## Neurologic Sequelae

Neurologic sequelae are mostly rare, but may result from mechanical or chemical injury. It may be due to misplaced spinal needle, surgical retractors, faulty positioning, pressure on peripheral nerves etc. Preexisting neurologic disease may also be exacerbated. Haematoma is usually associated with patients with clotting disorders. Contamination of local anaesthetics, needles or catheters may lead to abscess formation and septic meningitis. Aseptic meningitis can also occur. Direct neurotoxicity is extremely rare but chloroprocaine has some neurolytic actions. Preservatives of local anaesthetics may also be a factor.

Cauda equina syndrome may occur due to administration of hyperbaric local anaesthetics through subarachnoid catheters. Slow injection through narrow lumen catheter causes nonuniform distribution of local anaesthetic and exposure of unmyelinated nerve fibres to excessive high drug concentration. This causes adhesive arachnoiditis.

Direct neural trauma can occur from the needle or catheter.

All these complications should be properly recognised and may be confirmed by computed tomography or magnetic resonance imaging, whenever necessary.

## Failure/Inadequate Analgesia

Failure can occur due to inability to identify the subarachnoid space and lack of free-flow of CSF due to distorted anatomy, obesity, lack of experience on the part of anaesthetist, struggling patients, etc.

Inadequate analgesia may occur due to faulty selection of local anaesthetic, dose, vasoconstrictor, baricity, position, interspace and so on.

## Types of Spinal Anaesthesia

| | |
|---|---|
| 1. *Saddle block* | Upper level of analgesia $S_1$ Indications: Cystoscopy, surgery on perineum, anal surgery, etc. Lumbar puncture at $L_4$, $L_5$ on sitting position. |
| 2. *Low spinal* | Upper level of analgesia $L_1$, $T_{12}$ Perineal surgery, anal surgery, surgery on lower extremities, transurethral prostatectomy, etc. Lumbar puncture at $L_3$, $L_4$ on sitting or lateral position. |
| 3. *Medium spinal* | Upper level of analgesia $T_{10}$, $-T_8$ Lower abdominal surgery, repair of hernia, prostatectomy, hip surgery, etc. Lumbar puncture at $L_3$, $L_4$ on sitting or lateral position |
| 4. *High spinal* | Upper level of analgesia $T_4$ All abdominal surgery. Lumbar puncture at $L_2$ $L_3$ on lateral position. |
| 5. *Unilateral analgesia* | It is an attempt to minimise sympathetic block. But usually the block spreads bilaterally within a short time. |

## Density, Baricity and Patient Position

The density of cerebrospinal fluid at 37°C ranges from 1.001 to 1.005 g/ml. The density of a local anaesthetic solution is a function of its concentration and the fluid in which the drug is dissolved.

The baricity is expressed as the density of local anaesthetic solution divided by the density of CSF. It is the ratio between the two at the same temperature.

The local anaesthetic solutions can be of three types: hyperbaric, isobaric and hypobaric in relation to CSF.

1. *Hyperbaric:* Local anaesthetic solutions with densities greater than 1.008 g/ml at 37°C. Local anaesthetic solution in 5 to 8% dextrose are hyperbaric.

2. *Isobaric:* Local anaesthetic solutions with densities between 0.998 to 1.007 g/ml at 37°C. Local anaesthetics diluted with CSF or isotonic saline is isobaric.

3. *Hypobaric:* Local anaesthetic solutions with densities less than 0.997 g/ml at 37°C. It is prepared by diluting the local anaesthetic solution with water.

Distribution of local anaesthetic and level of anaesthesia mostly depends on the dose of local anaesthetic, baricity of the solution, and the posture of the patient during and immediately after spinal injection.

In lying supine position the highest point in the subarachnoid space is at the level of third lumbar (lumbar lordosis) and the lowest in the space is at the level of fifth thoracic (thoracic kyphosis). A hyperbaric solution will gravitate to the sacral and to the thoracic regions. In sitting position it may cause saddle block provided the position is kept for sometime after injection.

Hypobaric solutions tend to float in CSF and can be used in supine, lateral or in jack knife position. Head down tilt may help to limit the cephalad spread of the local anaesthetic solution in such cases.

Isobaric solutions tend to remain at the site of injection and produce the block. Commonly available local anaesthetic solution are made with normal saline and are isobaric. Common operations by using isobaric spinal block may include lower extremity, genitourinary, perineal and anal surgery.

## PROCEDURES FOR SPINAL ANAESTHESIA

A. *Equipment must be kept ready for spinal anaesthesia*

1. *Spinal kit:* A typical prepacked sterile disposable kit for spinal anaesthesia should include 22 or 25 gauze 10 cm long spinal needle, draping material, standard syringes and needles, 0.75% methyl paraben-free bupivacaine vial (hyperbaric), 1% lignocaine 10 mg/ml, vial of adrenaline 1 mg/ml lignocaine 4% (heavy).

2. Spinal anaesthesia may have significant cardiovascular and respiratory complications. Even sudden cardiac arrest may also occur. So resuscitation equipment and emergency drugs must be available.

3. Failure or inadequate analgesia may also occur and these cases may need general anaesthesia. Thus, anaesthesia machine, related equipment and drugs should always be there.

4. Monitoring equipment like pulse oximetry, BP instrument, etc. should be there.

5. Thus, spinal anaesthesia should be given in well equipped operation theatre with good operation table (with tilting arrangements) and good source of light.

6. A good assistant is needed to position the patient during spinal puncture.

B. *Preoperative visit is needed*

1. Proper selection of the patient is important.

2. Patient should be explained beforehand.

3. Assess the patient's physiological status particularly cardiovascular, respiratory and haematological condition. Skin condition of the back should be noted.

4. Obtain the valid consent of surgery and anaesthesia.
5. Obtain the investigation reports.

C. An IV drip should always by started before performing lumber puncture. Preloading with crystalline solution is necessary to prevent hypotension.

D. Proper positioning of the patient is needed. A good assistant may help in this matter. Lateral or sitting posture should be chosen according to the site of operation.

E. A full sterile technique should be adopted. Sterile gown and gloves should be worn. The skin is prepared with antiseptic lotion and draped in sterile condition. Spinal set should be opened and displayed

F. Selection of interspace for lumbar puncture. The spinal cord usually ends at the level of $L_2$. Spinal needle should be inserted below it usually at $L_3$ $L_4$ interlaminar space. The iliac crest usually lies at the level of $L_4$ (Fig. 4.5).

G. A small intradermal wheal of local anaesthetic is made at the selected space with a 25 gauge needle.

H. Selection of spinal needle is important. Either 22 or 25 gauge needle is used. A pencil point needle is preferred. Disposable introducer needles 18G may be used particularly when 25G spinal needle is used.

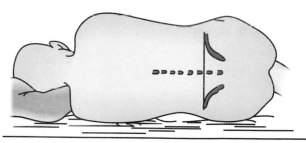

**Fig. 4.5:** Lateral position for spinal block

I. Selection of drug: Heavy lignocaine or bupivacaine is popularly used depending on approximate duration of operation. Isobaric or hypobaric solutions are also used as per indications.

J. The needle is carefully inserted in midline at $L_3-L_4$ or $L_4-L_5$ in lateral decubitus position of the patient keeping knees and head flexed on the chest. Sitting position may be used, if there is difficulty in separating the lumbar spinous processes or a low level of anaesthesia in intended.

K. The spinal needle is advanced with a little cephalad angle to pierce in the supraspinous ligament. Continued needle advancement pierces the ligamentum flavum and the dura mater. Needle placement in subarachnoid space is assumed by a distinct 'pop' felt by the fingers of the anaesthetist as the needle passes through the dura mater. It is further confirmed by the appearance of CSF at the hub. At this point the spinal needle should be correctly stabilised by the fingers. Then the syringe containing local anaesthetic solution is attached to the hub. Aspiration is done gently. If the CSF flow is clear, the local anaesthetic solution is gently introduced in the space. A rapid injection rate may push the anaesthetic toward higher dermatome levels. The syringe and needle are then removed as a single unit. The distance between the skin and subarachnoid space may vary from 3.5 to 5 cm (Fig. 4.6).

L. If blood tinged CSF flows, the needle should be removed and reinserted at a different interspace.

M. After removal of the needle and syringe, an antiseptic dressing should be given. Then the patient should be placed supine. Monitoring of pulse, respiration and blood pressure

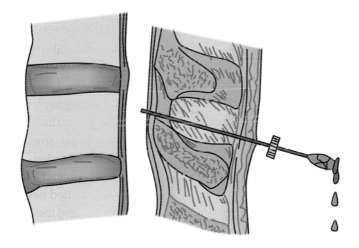

**Fig. 4.6:** Spinal needle in subarachnoid space

should be done for detection and treatment of any side effects, if any.

N. The distribution of block should be assessed. Sensory block can be ascertained by seeking response to pinprick or finger scratch. Motor block can be tested by asking the patient to raise the knees ($L_2$ $L_3$), to lift the leg, to dorsiflex the foot or to plantar flex the toes. When the sensory and motor block seem to be satisfactory, surgeon may be allowed to start the operation.

## CONTINUOUS SPINAL ANAESTHESIA

It is also known as catheter spinal anaesthesia. Here a catheter is introduced in subarachnoid space to administer local anaesthetic solution. It allows all the benefits of single injection spinal anaesthesia. But the added advantages include the prolongation of anaesthesia and control of the extent of block by adding the drug through the catheter, whenever needed.

The technique is usually simple and easy. A spinal preferably epidural needle is placed in subarachnoid space in the usual manner. The distance between the skin and the space is estimated. The catheter is then passed 3 cm into the subarachnoid space then the needle should be withdrawn gently over the catheter by well securing it firmly. The catheter should be 3 cm inside the space. Proper placement is confirmed by aspiration test and free flow of CSF.

Neurologic complications and postdural puncture headache are more common in this technique, Moreover, the advent of continuous epidural anaesthesia, the catheter spinal anaesthesia is not in vogue nowadays.

**Common Complications of Catheter Spinal Anaesthesia**

1. It may not be possible to thread the catheter beyond the needle bevel due to some anatomical reasons.
2. Breakage of catheter during insertion or removal can occur.
3. Knotting of the catheter in the space.
4. Catheter may be trapped by neural structures.
5. Catheter may be migrated into a blood vessel.
6. Catheter may be dislocated from the subarachnoid space resulting in epidural placement.
7. Cauda equina syndrome. It is mostly due to accumulation of large doses of local anaesthetic through a narrow lumen catheter. It causes adhesive arachnoiditis.

# SPINAL NEUROLYTIC BLOCK

Here small amounts of neurolytic agent like alcohol or phenol are introduced into the subarachnoid space to denervate large parts of the body. These blocks usually cause destruction of the posterior root ganglion. It may be theoretically possible to produce selective sensory block and spare motor power and sphincter function.

It is usually indicated to alleviate persistent chronic pain particularly in patients with short life expectancy as in cases of terminal cancer. Neurolytic block should be attempted when all other measures of pain relief fail.

Ethyl alcohol in absolute concentrations is used for subarachnoid neurolytic block. Weaker solution can be used to produce selective destruction of smaller sensory fibres. Alcohol is hypobaric in CSF. It causes intense pain with injection but neurolysis is prompt.

Phenol in glycerine produces no pain on injection and onset of neurolysis is delayed. It is hyperbaric in CSF. Ten per cent phenol solution is predictably neurolytic.

## Technique

With hypobaric alcohol, the spinal segments to be blocked should be positioned upper most in relation to other segments. But with hyperbaric phenol the position should be reversed.

Initially a very small amount of neurolytic agent should be used to note the effect prior to proceeding with further injections. The extent of effect should be tested frequently to avoid extensive spread. Patient movement during or immediately after injection can cause unwanted spread of block.

Usual preparations and precautions should be made as with spinal anaesthesia. The patient is positioned in lateral position with affected side uppermost. Subarachnoid puncture should be done in the usual manner at the appropriate interspace. About 2 ml of CSF should be withdrawn and then exactly 0.5 ml of alcohol is injected slowly. Patient should then be placed prone with 5° head down position. The position should be maintained for about 30 minutes to produce the effect.

# CHAPTER 5

# Epidural Anaesthesia

## INTRODUCTION

Epidural anaesthesia is obtained by blocking spinal nerve roots as they emerge from the spinal cord and traverse the epidural (peridural or extradural) space. Local anaesthetic solution is deposited outside the dura and the block can be performed in the sacral, lumbar, thoracic or cervical regions. The commonest popular route is lumbar and it is known as lumbar epidural block. Sacral epidural block is known as caudal block. Anaesthesia occurs slowly and develops in a segmental manner.

## ANATOMY

The epidural space is a circular space surrounding the dural sac and all its extensions. It lies from the foramen magnum to the coccyx. The potential space exists between the lining of vertebral canal and the dural sac. It is more extensive and easily distensible posteriorly. Anteriorly the dura closely adheres to the periosteum of vertebral bodies. Laterally there are intervertebral foramina and vertebral pedicles. Lateral extension of the epidural space accompany the spinal nerves through the intervertebral foramina into the paravertebral space. Anatomically there is free communication of epidural space with the paravertebral space.

The space contains areolar tissue, loose fat and spinal nerve roots with their dural sleeves. Spinal arteries and a venous plexus are also present. The cavity has a fluid capacity of approximately 25 ml. Fluid injected into the sacral or lumbar epidural space may spread upto foramen magnum and laterally through intervertebral foramina.

Due to the lateral extension of the extradural space through intervertebral foramina, any change of intrathoracic pressure is reflected within the extradural space. The negative intrathoracic pressure is transmitted to the extradural space. These pressure changes are most marked in thoracic region but may extend down to the lumbar area.

The extradural negative pressure varies with the depth of respiration and in fact, with the intrapleural pressure.

- During epidural injection in a midline sagittal plane, the following structures are pierced:
  1. Skin and subcutaneous tissue
  2. Supraspinous ligament
  3. Interspinous ligament
  4. Ligamentum flavum.

## SITE OF ACTION OF LOCAL ANAESTHETIC

1. On the spinal nerves as they traverse epidural space.
2. On the nerves as they pass out through intervertebral foramina.
3. On the nerves in subarachnoid space. It is said that the local anaesthetic may reach in variable amount in subarachnoid space by diffusion.

## FACTORS CONTROLLING THE EXTENT OF ANAESTHESIA

1. Volume of the solution
2. Dose and concentration of drug
3. Selection of proper local anaesthetic
4. Selection of appropriate interspace

5. Speed of injection
6. Position of the patient
7. Effect of gravity
8. Specific gravity of the local anaesthetic solution.

## Some Clinical Factors may affect the Epidural Spread

1. Spread is greater in the elderly. A relatively small amount is needed to produce the same extent of anaesthesia.
2. Spread is greater in pregnant mothers.
3. In arteriosclerosis and occlusive arterial disease the spread is greater than in normal subjects.
4. Spread is decreased in shock, dehydration, etc.
5. A greater dose is needed in taller patients.

## EPIDURAL BLOCK

### Physiological Effects of Epidural Block

The physiological effects of epidural block are mostly similar to those of subarachnoid block. These are discussed in the previous chapter. But some differences may be observed mostly due to use of large volumes of local anaesthetic solution in epidural block and significant systemic absorption of the drug. These effects are more pronounced when combined with adrenaline. Severe myocardial depression may occur particularly in presence of hypovolaemia.

### Indications of Epidural Block

1. Epidural anaesthesia may be benefitted in certain circumstances
   (a) Poor risk patients
   (b) Cardiac diseases

(c) Respiratory diseases

(d) Metabolic derangements

(e) When spinal anaesthesia is more problematic.

(f) When general anaesthesia is contraindicated.

In these cases all the merits and demerits of epidural anaesthesia should be judged and balanced to get the better outcome.

2. Chronic pain relief

3. Postoperative pain relief

4. Obstetric pain relief

5. To produce contraction of gut

6. To reduce blood loss during pelvic surgery

## Contraindications of Epidural Block

1. Severe shock, haemorrhage

2. Unwilling, noncooperative patients

3. Patient wants to remain unconscious during operation

4. Coagulation disorders

5. Skin condition infected at the site of injection

6. Patients with previous laminectomy

7. Valid consent is not available.

## Uses of Epidural Block

1. As a sole technique in various operations abdominal, pelvic, anal, rectal, lower extremity, chronic pain syndrome.

2. In combination with IV drugs.

3. In combination with general anaesthesia

4. Continuous epidural analgesia for painless labour.

5. Epidural opioid in chronic pain syndromes, in management of chest injury with fractured ribs.

## Advantages of Epidural Analgesia

1. Region of anaesthesia is mostly well marked.
2. Duration of anaesthesia can be prolonged with catheter technique.
3. Neurologic injury is less.
4. Postdural puncture headache minimised.
5. Nausea/vomiting minimal.
6. Urinary retention is less.

## Disadvantages of Epidural Anaesthesia

1. The technique needs extra skill and experience.
2. Muscle relaxation may not be complete.
3. Large volume of local anaesthetic is needed and thus may increase the incidence of toxic reactions.
4. Inadvertent dural puncture can occur.
5. Catheter technique may induce injury to venous plexus.
6. Incomplete segmental block may occur.
7. Backache may be frequent.

## Epidural Anaesthesia Kit

It is a prepacked sterile disposable kit for epidural anaesthesia. It should contain:

1. Long Tuohy needle
2. Epidural catheter with stylet and distal marking in cm.
3. Catheter or syringe adaptor.
4. 0.2 μm pore size bacterial filter
5. Preservative–free local anaesthetic solution
6. Standard syringe and needles, lignocaine vial, saline for infiltration anaesthesia.
7. Sterile dressing and draping material.

## Technique of Lumbar Epidural Block

1. Preanaesthetic check-up is essential.
   (a) Selection of the patient should be done carefully.
   (b) Proper assessment of cardiovascular, respiratory and metabolic and haematological status.
   (c) Skin condition of puncture site should be examined.
   (d) Inform and explain the patient about the technique.
   (e) Obtain valid consent for anaesthesia and operation.
2. Epidural block should be done in well equipped operation theatre. Anaesthesia machine and equipment, monitoring devices, resuscitation equipment and emergency drugs should be available.
3. Sterilised epidural kit should be there.
4. An intravenous infusion with indwelling cannula must be started before the procedure.
5. Correct positioning is essential. A good assistant is always helpful. Lateral decubitus or sitting position is usually adopted. The lateral position with knees and head flexed on the chest is useful.
6. The skin of the back is prepared with antiseptic lotion and draped as usual. Operator must wear sterile gown and gloves with usual precautions.
7. A local anaesthetic skin wheal is made at the selected lumbar interspace. Appropriate long Tuohy needle (with a curved distal end) is inserted gently until it is engaged in the spinal ligaments.
8. The stylet is then removed and an air or liquid filled syringe with well movable proper plunger is attached to the needle: The epidural needle is advanced slowly in 2 mm increments.

The plunger of the syringe is depressed intermittently. If the tip of the needle is in the ligaments, the plunger can not be depressed smoothly and it bounces back. But when the tip is in the epidural space, there is feeling of loss of resistance. Then the plunger can be depressed and it does not bounce back.

Alternatively, if a drop of sterile liquid is placed in the open needle hub, the fluid is sucked in by the negative pressure of epidural space.

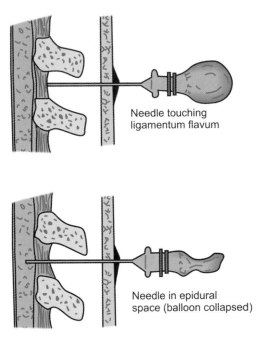

Needle touching
ligamentum flavum

Needle in epidural
space (balloon collapsed)

**Fig. 5.1:** Detection of epidural space (balloon technique)

*Note:* Odom's indicator and Macintosh balloon techniques (Fig. 5.1) are previously used to detect the presence of negative pressure in epidural space. But the loss of resistance test seems to be easy and reliable for identification of the space.

9. Once the needle is in the epidural space the local anaesthetic solution is injected gently after negative aspiration test.

   When the needle is in epidural space, the bevel of the needle should be directed appropriately to distribute the solution either caudal or cranial as needed.

   • *Aspiration Test:* When needle is in epidural space, a syringe is attached to the needle and by gentle aspiration, evidence of CSF or blood is noted. If there is neither CSF nor blood, the operator should inject the local anaesthetic solution. If blood or CSF is found the technique may be abandoned or another interspace may be selected.

10. Local anaesthetic solution should be injected fractionally. After injection the needle and stylet should be taken out together. The injection site is then dressed.

11. Position of the patient after injection: It is said that head down position at 10° tilt for upper abdominal surgery, supine horizontal posture for lower abdominal surgery and head up tilt at 5° for perineal surgery may be beneficial.

12. *Continuous epidural technique:*

    When the tip of the needle is in the epidural space, a plastic epidural catheter with or without stylet is passed 2 to 3 cm into the epidural space. The epidural needle is then removed over the catheter. It should be noted that the catheter must not be withdrawn through the epidural needle as it may tear and remain in the space.

The catheter should be secured with adhesive tape. A syringe adaptor with a bacterial filter should be attached to the proximal end of the epidural catheter.

After the end of surgery the catheter is removed gently and proper dressing should be done. It must be examined that the catheter is removed intact and it should be recorded in the anaesthetic chart.

Continuous epidural technique is indicated when prolonged anaesthesia is needed.

Unilateral block or absence of analgesia can occur if the long epidural catheter is misplaced far away so as to pass out through the intervertebral foramina.

Epidural catheter aspiration may be risky as extradural veins are fragile and may rupture or collapse due to large degree of suction.

13. *Common local anaesthetics for epidural anaesthesia:*
    (a) Lignocaine 1 to 2%, onset of action ranges from 5 to 15 min; duration of action ranges from 1 hour to 2 hours.
    (b) Bupivacaine 0.25 to 0.75%, onset of action ranges from 10 to 20 min. Duration of action ranges from 2 to 4 hours. Bupivacaine 0.75% solution is recommended for surgical procedure, but not in obstetrics. Requirement of local anaesthetics in pregnancy is usually less than that of nonpregnant patients.
    (c) Mepivacaine 1.5%.
    (d) Etidocaine 1%.

- *Note:* The addition of adrenaline 5 µg/ml to local anaesthetics for epidural anaesthesia prolongs their effect, reduces their blood concentration, lessens the risk of systemic toxicity.

## COMPLICATIONS OF EPIDURAL ANAESTHESIA

Complications of epidural block are mostly similar to those of spinal block with the added risk of inadvertent dural puncture and systemic toxicity of local anaesthetics.

1. *Accidental dural puncture:* It may lead to (A) total spinal anaesthesia, (B) postspinal headache.

   A *Total spinal anaesthesia:* Accidental injection of large volume of local anaesthetic in subarachnoid space may pass cephalad in cerebrospinal fluid. It may cause respiratory failure due to paralysis of phrenic nerve and direct medullary depression. There may be severe hypotension and cardiovascular collapse. Convulsion can occur by systemic absorption of the drug and by direct spread in CSF.

   - *Management:* Operator should be extremely cautious in performing the epidural block. He should detect the epidural space and careful aspiration test should be done. If CSF comes through the needle, he may convert it to spinal anaesthesia or choose another interspace for epidural block. A subarachnoid catheter may be passed to provide continuous spinal anaesthesia.

     Early recognition and rapid resuscitory measures are needed. Skilled rapid resuscitation is always followed by complete recovery. There may not be any need to cancel the operation.

(a) Resuscitation equipment and emergency drugs should be available. Anaesthetic machine and equipment should also be available.

(b) Intravenous infusion is essential.

(c) Vasopressors

(d) Diazepam may be needed to treat convulsion.

(e) Endotracheal intubation, IPPV, adequate oxygenation.

(f) Several hours may be needed in complete recovery.

B. *Postspinal headache:* Usually a large bore needle (16 or 18 G) is used to perform epidural block. Thus, if dural tap occurs, the gap seems to be of considerable size to leak CSF and cause postspinal headache.

Postspinal headache can be managed in the following order:

(a) Bed rest. No ambulation.

(b) Analgesics

(c) Intake of large volumes of fluid, IV or oral

(d) Extradural infusion of sterile saline.

(e) Epidural blood patch: 15 to 20 ml of autologous blood is injected in epidural space with full aseptic precautions.

2. *Systemic toxicity of local anaesthetics. Prevention can be tried with the following*:

(a) Appropriate use of test doses.

(b) Aspiration test prior to injection of local anaesthetic.

(c) Addition of adrenaline lessens the risk of toxicity. Management is already discussed in the chapter of Spinal Anaesthesia.

3. *Hypotension*: It may be due to systemic absorption of local anaesthetic drug, high sympathetic block and bradycardia due to sympathetic block to $T_1-T_4$.
4. Respiratory depression
5. Inadvertent contamination of chemical irritants
6. Haematoma formation. It may occur in patients with coagulation disorders or with anticoagulants
7. Epidural abscess
8. Injury to spinal cord and nerve roots
9. Prolonged analgesia or paraesthesia
10. Incomplete block/failure.

## SPINAL/EPIDURAL ANAESTHESIA FOR CAESAREAN SECTION

### Advantages

1. It permits the mother to remain awake during delivery.
2. Reduces the risk of maternal aspiration.
3. Minimises the risk of neonatal drug depression.
4. Spinal anaesthesia is technically easy to perform and provides reliable and rapid anaesthesia. Epidural anaesthesia is technically more difficult to perform. It can be applied to both labour and caesarean delivery. But it is time consuming and potential for local anaesthetic toxicity.

### Contraindications of Epidural Anaesthesia

#### *Absolute*

1. Infection at the site of injection
2. Severe hypovolaemia, dehydration

3. Raised intracranial pressure
4. Coagulation abnormalities
5. Patient refusal

*Relative*

1. Neurologic disease
2. History of back surgery
3. History of back pain
4. Systemic infection

## PRE-ECLAMPSIA AND EPIDURAL ANAESTHESIA

Epidural anaesthesia may be beneficial for the patient with pre-eclampsia in certain aspects:

1. It can reduce hyperventilation by decreasing and allaying the pain sensation.
2. It reduces catecholamine release due to pain.
3. It allays fear, anxiety and tension.
4. It can improve uteroplacental blood flow.
5. Continuous lumbar epidural anaesthesia may be helpful for vaginal delivery of pre-eclamptic parturient. Initially a segmental block ($T_{10}$–$T_{11}$) will provide analgesia for uterine contractions. At the second stage the anaesthesia can be extended to provide perineal anaesthesia.
6. Caesarean section can be safely done with epidural block. But before that blood pressure must be controlled, adequate hydration is needed and coagulation status must be normal. Continuous monitoring of intraarterial pressure, urine output, CVP and foetal heart rate is useful.

# CHAPTER 6

# Caudal
# Anaesthesia

## INTRODUCTION

Caudal anaesthesia is a particular form of epidural anaesthesia where the access of the space is made through the sacral hiatus. It is actually the sacral epidural block. It is very suitable for block of the sacral and lumbar nerves.

## ANATOMY

Sacrum is a large triangular bone formed by the fusion of the five sacral vertebrae. It articulates with the fifth lumbar vertebra above, the ileac bone laterally and the coccyx below. Pelvic surface is concave from above downwards and from side to side. It supports various structures like ileac vessels, rectum etc. Posterior surface is convex and rough and in the midline from above downward is the sacral crest with its 3 or 4 rudimentary spinous processes. The failure of fusion of the lamina of the fifth and sometimes of fourth results in sacral hiatus. It communicates with the sacral part of vertebral canal. Lateral surfaces are broader and articulate with ileum.

The hiatus is usually V or U shaped notch and the unfused lamina of each side form bony prominences known as cornua. The hiatus is covered by sacrococcygeal ligament which is formed from the supraspinous ligament, the interspinous ligament and the ligamentum flavum. It is pierced by coccygeal and fifth sacral nerves. It is above the sacrococcygeal junction, usually 4 to 5 cm from the lip of coccyx.

### Sacral Canal

Sacral canal runs throughout the length of the bone. Above it is continuous with the lumbar vertebral canal. Its lower end is the sacral hiatus closed by posterior sacrococcygeal membrane. Some fibrous bands may be there and the space may thus be divided into compartments. On each lateral wall of the canal four foramina are present. Average capacity of the sacral canal is about 32 to 34 ml. Its average length is 3 to 4 cm.

Sacral canal contains the following:

1. Dural sac: It ends at lower border of $S_2$ in the adult. Piamater continues as filum terminale.
2. Sacral nerves and coccygeal nerves with their dorsal root ganglion. Each sacral nerve is ensheathed from the dura.
3. Venous plexus
4. Areolar tissue, fatty tissue

Sacral canal is triangular in shape on cross-section. The canal is often referred to as the caudal canal and it is a part of epidural space (Fig. 6.1).

The dural sac almost fills the vertebral canal except the epidural space. It ends between $S_1$ and $S_2$. The vertebral canal ends at the sacral hiatus. The average distance between the apex of hiatus and the dural sac is about 47 mm. The hiatus is covered by the sacrococcygeal ligament.

Anatomical anomalies of the sacrum is common. Some of them are as follows:

1. Dural sac may extend below the middle of $S_2$.
2. Apex of sacral hiatus may lie superior to the lower third of $S_4$.
3. Large deficiencies in the posterior wall.
4. Narrowed anteroposterior diameter at the apex of hiatus.
5. Absence of hiatus
6. Bony blocks of the sacral canal.

*Note*:

1. Local anaesthetic solution injected in the sacral canal passes upwards in the epidural space depending on:
   (a) volume of injection fluid
   (b) force of injection
   (c) degree of leakage through intervertebral foramina.
   (d) consistency of epidural space.

2. The epidural space communicates with the paravertebral spaces, as a result the extradural block may affect:
   (a) anterior and posterior nerve roots
   (b) mixed spinal nerves
   (c) sympathetic chain ganglia
   (d) grey and white rami communicates
   (e) visceral afferent fibres accompanying the sympathetic fibres.

## PHYSIOLOGY OF CAUDAL BLOCK

1. Anaesthesia usually occurs slowly. Onset of anaesthesia is about 5 min. Maximum extent and intensity is expected at about 20 min after injection.
2. Sensory loss is mostly satisfactory. Muscular relaxation may be inadequate.
3. Cardiovascular alterations are minimal.
4. Respiration is not much affected.
5. Gastrointestinal tone may be increased.

## INDICATIONS OF CAUDAL BLOCK

Caudal anaesthesia may be helpful in various surgical procedures. But it does not provide adequate muscular relaxation. Thus, it is not much helpful in intra-abdominal procedures. However, it can be satisfactorily used in the following procedures:

1. Anal surgery, rectal surgery, cystoscopy.
2. Haemorrhoidectomies, gynaecological, perineal operations.
3. Obstetric delivery, forceps delivery.
4. Management of chronic pain syndromes in pelvis and lower extremities.
5. In diagnostic and therapeutic purposes: low backache, sciatica, vasospastic disease, pelvic pain, etc.
6. In paediatric surgery: circumcision, hernia repair, anal and rectal surgery.
7. Postoperative pain relief.
8. Prolonged post-traumatic pain relief.
9. To control eclamspsia.
10. To treat renal colic, to relieve anuria and oliguria associated with reflex renal ischaemia.

## CONTRAINDICATIONS OF CAUDAL BLOCK

1. Infection at the injection site
2. Pilonidal cyst
3. Sacral anomalies
4. Obesity
5. Central nervous system disorders
6. Unwilling, uncooperative patients
7. Susceptibility to local anaesthetics.

## ADVANTAGES OF CAUDAL ANAESTHESIA

1. Incidence of headache is minimised.
2. Cardiovascular depression is less.

3. Provides postoperative analgesia.
4. Location of the sacral hiatus and technique of caudal block are technically easy in children.

## DISADVANTAGES OF CAUDAL ANAESTHESIA

1. Onset of anaesthesia is slow
2. Extent of analgesia may not be accurately controlled
3. Muscular relaxation is inadequate
4. Technically difficult in adult patients
5. Accidental subarachnoid injection is possible
6. Systemic toxicity with local anaesthetic can occur
7. Risk of intravascular injection is there
8. Large volumes of local anaesthetic are used
9. Anatomical anomalies may cause technical difficulty and thus failures are common
10. Risk of infection
11. Constant supervision is needed
12. Trauma to periosteum and bony structures.

## TECHNIQUE OF CAUDAL BLOCK (FIGS 6.1 AND 6.2) (COLLINS, 1972)

Caudal anaesthesia can be instituted with the patient in lateral, prone or jack knife position. Prone position is preferred.

Proper aseptic precautions are needed. After sterile skin preparation and draping, the posterior superior iliac spine, sacral cornua and sacral hiatus are identified. The sacral hiatus is at about 5 cm from the tip of coccyx between the cornua. The skin at the site of injection is infiltrated with local anaesthetic in the usual manner.

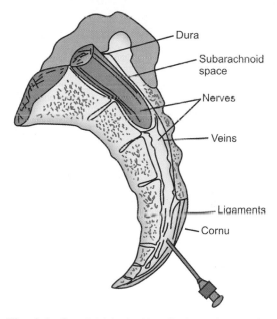

Dura

Subarachnoid space

Nerves

Veins

Ligaments

Cornu

**Fig. 6.1:** Caudal block. Needle just pierces the sacrococcygeal ligament

A needle is inserted perpendicular to the skin surface until the needle tip contacts the sacrum in sacral canal. The needle is then withdrawn a little from the periosteum. The hub of the needle is depressed 10 to 15 degrees and then gently advanced about 2 cm into the caudal canal.

The placement of the needle in the caudal canal below the dural sac should be confirmed. Aspiration test should always be routine. It will indicate no flow of blood or CSF. A 5 ml of air is injected through the needle and there will be no feeling of crepitus on the skin over the needle tip. Intravenous or

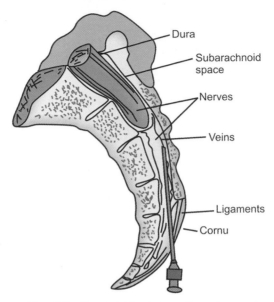

**Fig. 6.2:** Caudal block (needle advanced upto below the level of S$_2$ vertebra)

subanachnoid injection of large volume of local anaesthetic is sometimes fatal.

Then the anaesthetic solution can be injected gently into the caudal space. If needed, a catheter may also be introduced through a large bore needle and allowed to remain in place. Then the needle is removed over the catheter. Appropriate connections are made to the free end catheter (adaptors, syringe, needle) for administration of local anaesthetic. It is the catheter technique used for continuous caudal anaesthesia (Fig. 6.3).

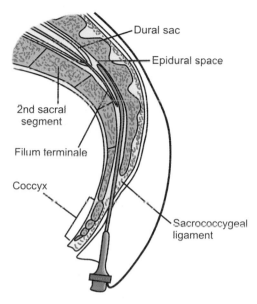

**Fig. 6.3:** Caudal analgesia. Catheter in caudal space

Level of anaesthesia must be properly checked every 15 minutes interval. Continuous monitoring of vital signs is always needed to detect any adverse effects.

The correct position of the caudal needle or catheter should indicate:

1. Onset of analgesia and loss of sensation within 10 minutes after injection.
2. No CSF or blood in aspiration test.
3. No crepitus or palpable swelling superficial to sacrum.
4. Progressive spread of anaesthesia.

5. Evidence of sympathetic block such as vasodilatation, flushing, cessation of sweating.

6. Relief of abdominal uterine cramps in obstetric patients.

## COMPLICATIONS OF CAUDAL ANAESTHESIA

As caudal anaesthesia is a form of epidural anaesthesia, complications are mostly similar.

1. Subarachnoid injection, Massive spinal anaesthesia
2. Hypotension
3. Intravascular injection
4. Systemic toxic effects of local anaesthetics
5. Technical complications: Breakage of needle, tear of catheter, injury of nerve fibres
6. Infection of the coccyx, sacrum, epidural space.

## DANGERS OF CONTINUOUS CAUDAL ANALGESIA IN OBSTETRIC PATIENTS

1. Foetal hypoxia may occur due to maternal hypotension.
2. High spread of anaesthesia may cause prolonged or arrested labour.
3. Incidence of operative deliveries may be increased.
4. Usual complications of caudal analgesia like massive spinal anaesthesia, systemic toxicity of local anaesthetics etc. may also limit the use of caudal anaesthesia in obstetrics.

- However, caudal anaesthesia may have some beneficial effect in certain obstetric cases:
  1. Patients with toxaemia
  2. In premature labour

3. Patients with cardiac, pulmonary, renal or metabolic disorders.
4. For forceps delivery.
5. In emergency caesarean section in patients with full stomach.

- Therapeutic indications of caudal analgesia/anaesthesia:
  1. Eclampsia
  2. Oliguria/anuria, renal colic
  3. Postoperative pain relief
  4. Postoperative paralytic ileus
  5. Arterial embolism in lower extremities
  6. Vasospastic diseases of legs
  7. Chronic cold feet
  8. Diabetic neuropathy

- *Note:* Caudal block is not much popular nowadays due to high incidence of failure rates mostly due to anatomical anomalies of the sacrum. However, the technique seems to be useful in children as the landmarks can be identified easily.

# CHAPTER 7

# Intravenous Regional Anaesthesia

## INTRODUCTION

Intravenous regional anaesthesia involves the technique of anaesthesia of a limb by injection of large volumes of local anaesthetic solution intravenously while the limb has been made ischaemic by a tourniquet. It is also known as Bier block after the name A. Bier. In August 1908, Bier described the method and established the effectiveness of local anaesthetics administered intravenously and localised by tourniquet to produce effective regional anaesthesia (Fig. 7.1).

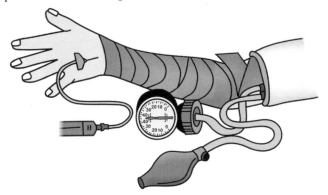

**Fig. 7.1:** Intravenous regional anaesthesia

## MECHANISM OF ACTION

Local anaesthetics administered IV produce vasodilation acting directly on vessel walls. The drug also diffuses into the tissues, produces block of small nerve fibres and nerve endings and causes analgesia/anaesthesia.

Localisation of the local anaesthetic agent to the particular limb is most important. To achieve this objective, certain steps are usually followed:

1. The limb must be produced ischaemic by using an Esmarch bandage.
2. Tourniquet must be applied to prevent entry of blood.
3. A large volume of dilute solution of local anaesthetic should be injected distal to the tourniquet. The volume of the solution must be enough to fill the vascular bed of the limb and the concentration of local anaesthetic must be adequate to produce satisfactory anaesthesia. The dose should not exceed the maximum safe dose limit for the risk of systemic toxicity.

## ADVANTAGES

1. The technique is easy and simple and requires little technical skill.
2. It may be used in various procedures on the limbs such as treatment of fractures, muscle injury, tendon injury, etc.
3. It is extremely predictable method.
4. It can be used in all age groups including children.
5. Onset of action is rapid. Surgical anaesthesia is usually within 10 minutes.
6. Muscle relaxation is profound.
7. Recovery is rapid.
8. Little or no intraoperative sedation or analgesia is required.

## DISADVANTAGES

1. *Risk of systemic toxicity:* Prevention can be attempted with the use of smaller doses and low concentrations of local anaesthetic within the range of effectiveness and by careful release of tourniquet.

2. The use of the technique is limited to limb surgery.
3. It is not much helpful for prolonged surgery.
4. It requires continuous vigilance at all times.

## INDICATIONS

1. To provide analgesia/anaesthesia in extremities.
2. Procedure of upper extremity below the elbow and distal lower extremity.
3. For ganglion excision, trigger finger repair, removal of foreign bodies and carpal tunnel syndrome, manipulation of fractures, etc.

## CONTRAINDICATIONS

1. History of drug sensitivity to local anaesthetics.
2. Patients with liver diseases, cardiac patients and patients with deficient peripheral circulation.
3. In debilitated, malnourished patients.
4. In myasthenia gravis.

## TECHNIQUE OF INTRAVENOUS REGIONAL ANAESTHESIA

An intravenous catheter is inserted in a distal portion of the involved extremity usually on the dorsum of the hand or foot and it is to be attached to a syringe through an extension tube for injection of the local anaesthetic solution.

A double pneumatic tourniquet is applied proximally and the limb is elevated to reduce its blood content. However, this can be done more efficiently by applying Esmarch bandage to exsanguinate the limb. Esmarch bandage should be wrapped tightly from the distal end to complete the exsanguination.

The distal tourniquet is then inflated followed by the proximal tourniquet, both to about 100 mm Hg above the patient's systolic pressure. The distal tourniquet is then released. This procedure helps to eliminate tourniquet pain. Now the limb shows mottled and cadaveric appearances after the removal of elastic bandage.

Then the local anaesthetic solution preferably 0.5% lignocaine without adrenaline is injected slowly through the IV catheter. Usually 25 to 50 ml is needed for upper extremity and from 100 to 200 ml for lower extremity. Care should be taken that the dose of lignocaine should not exceed 3 mg/kg.

Chloroprocaine is not suitable for intravenous regional anaesthesia as it may cause thrombophlebitis. Bupivacaine is also avoided due to its systemic toxic effects.

Onset of anaesthesia is mostly rapid and duration of anaesthesia ranges from 45 to 60 minutes. Initially the patient feels warmth and tingling of the limb and gradually the muscular paralysis becomes evident.

When the tourniquet pain will appear, the distal tourniquet can be inflated and then deflating the proximal tourniquet. It can extend the duration of anaesthesia a little longer.

At the end of operation the tourniquet is released. There is return of circulation and the local anaesthetic is washed out into the systemic circulation. As a result sensation and muscular tone return within a few minutes.

## COMPLICATIONS

1. *Systemic toxicity*: It may be due to sudden release or premature deflation of the tourniquet. It may be

characterized by drowsiness, bradycardia, hypotension and ECG absormalities. Early detection and careful management is essential. IV fluids, vasopressor and appropriate resuscitation are needed. Slow or intermittent deflations and inflations of the tourniquet at the end of surgery is recommended to prevent excessive blood concentrations of local anaesthetic. Limb movement should be restricted after release of tourniquet to minimise anaesthetic blood levels.

2. Methaemoglobinaemia may occur if prilocaine is used. Total dose of prilocaine should not exceed 600 mg in adults. However, rapid metabolism of prilocaine may minimise the risk of systemic toxicity.

# CHAPTER 8

# Nerve Blocks

## BLOCKS OF HEAD AND NECK

### Field Block of Scalp (Fig. 8.1)

*Anatomy*

A large number of nerves take part in cutaneous supply of the head and neck.

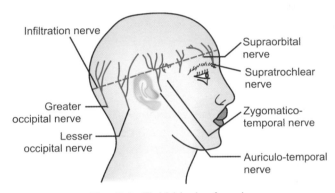

**Fig. 8.1:** Field block of scalp

The trigeminal nerve innervates anterior two-third of the scalp and face and the posterior two-third is supplied by the posterior divisions of cervical nerves. The trigeminal nerve has three divisions, ophthalmic, maxillary and mandibular nerves. There are four sensory nerves in front of ear namely:

1. Supratrochlear nerve from ophthalmic division
2. Supraorbital nerve from ophthalmic division
3. Zygomatico-temporal nerve from maxillary division
4. Auriculotemporal nerve from mandibular division.

There are four sensory nerves behind the ear from the cervical plexus.

1. Greater auricular nerve
2. Greater occipital nerve
3. Lesser occipital nerve
4. Least occipital nerve

All these nerves travel upwards to converge towards the vertex of scalp.

Besides these sensory nerves, one motor nerve temporal branch of facial nerve is in front of the ear and another motor nerve, posterior auricular branch of facial nerve lie behind the ear.

### Technique

A line of infiltration passing through the glabella and occiput encircling the head should be done to block the whole scalp. The injections must be intradermal, subcutaneous, intramuscular and periosteal up to the bone. This will block all the nerves.

However, appropriate rhomboid injections around the operative site may be another easy alternative technique.

### Indications

1. Sebaceous cyst removal
2. Small cuts and wounds repair.

### Greater and Lesser Occipital Nerve Block

A line is drawn between the occipital protuberance and the mastoid process. A needle is inserted about 2 cm lateral to occipital protuberance in the subcutaneous layer and the injection is made along the line and then directed towards the mastoid process to deposit another 3 to 4 ml of the anaesthetic solution. Both the nerves will be blocked.

## Greater Auricular Nerve Block

This nerve can be easily blocked by subcutaneous infiltration of about 10 ml of the local anaesthetic solution along the posterior aspect of the mastoid process.

## Auriculotemporal Nerve Block

The nerve is located superior to the temporomandibular joint along with superficial temporal artery. A skin wheal is made between the pulsation of artery and the tragus just at temporomandibular joint. A needle is passed through the wheal perpendicular to skin. After negative aspiration test, about 5 ml of the local anaesthetic solution is injected to block the nerve.

## Trigeminal Nerve Block

Trigeminal nerve is the **sensory nerve** of the face and front half of the scalp and **motor nerve** to the muscles of mastication except buccinator. The fifth cranial nerve has 5 ganglia on it.

1. The semilunar or Gasserian ganglion on nerve trunk
2. Ciliary ganglion on ophthalmic division
3. Sphenopalatine ganglion on maxillary division
4. Otic ganglion on mandibular division
5. Submaxillary or Langley's ganglion on mandibular division.

## Gasserian Ganglion Block

*Gasserian ganglion* corresponds to the ganglion on the posterior root of a spinal nerve. It is a large oval ganglion lying within the cranium in a dural capsule. It is accessible through the foramen ovale which lies at the base of lateral pterygoid plate. The smooth infratemporal plane is anterior to foramen ovale.

## Technique

The patient may lie supine or sit. Patient looks straight. A point is taken 3 cm from the angle of mouth at a level of second upper molar tooth. A skin wheal is done there. The midpoint of zygomatic arch is marked. Noting the line of intersection of two planes, one from skin wheal at the corner of mouth and midpoint of zygoma and the other passing through skin wheal to the pupil of eye, the needle is directed towards the midpoint of zygoma to strike the infratemporal plane. It is directed till the contact of infratemporal plane is lost and then the needle is advanced 1 to 1.5 cm to reach the foramen ovale.

Paraesthesia may occur radiating to lower jaw. The local anaesthetic solution may be deposited gently.

### Indications

1. Trigeminal neuralgia
2. Alcohol/phenol injection for permanent pain relief
3. Pain due to malignant disease or post herpetic neuralgia.

### Complications

1. Paraesthetic pain
2. Dry tearless eye, corneal ulcer
3. Inadvertent subdural injection.

### Maxillary Nerve Block (Fig. 8.2)

The maxillary nerve is one of the main branches of trigeminal nerve. It can be blocked after it leaves the middle cranial fossa through the foramen rotundum. It comes to lie in the pterygopalatine fossa between the skull and upper jaw. The nerve can be blocked at this location by an approach across the infratemporal fossa. The sphenopalatine ganglion is located in pterygopalatine fossa. Blocking of the nerve will produce analgesia in an area that includes the upper jaw and its derivatives including the skin of the upper lip, side of the nose, lower eyelid and malar region, the teeth of upper jaw, etc.

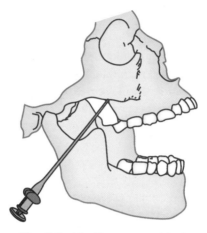

**Fig. 8.2:** Maxillary nerve block

*Indications*

1. Tic douloureux
2. Malignancy maxillary region
3. Surgery of maxillary sinus
4. Dental procedures in upper jaw.

*Technique*

A wheal is raised below the midpoint of zygomatic arch. The needle is introduced through it at the coronoid notch of the mandible. It is gently advanced across the infratemporal fossa until it strikes the lateral pterygoid plate at a depth of about

4 cm. The needle is walked anteriorly along the lateral pterygoid plate and advanced until it reaches the pterygopalatine fossa. It is further advanced for about 1 cm and the anaesthetic solution (lignocaine 1.5% 3 ml) is deposited after the negative aspiration test.

*Complications*

1. Haemorrhage due to puncture of terminal branches of maxillary artery
2. Intraneural injection
3. Spread of local anaesthetics to optic nerve.
4. Transient paralysis of the sixth cranial nerve.

## Mandibular Nerve Block (Fig. 8.3)

The mandibular nerve is the largest branch of trigeminal nerve. It leaves the skull through the foramen ovale in the middle cranial fossa. It passes immediately posterior to the lateral pterygoid plate of the sphenoid bone and between the pterygoid muscles. It supplies the mandible, pharynx, lower teeth, anterior two-third of the tongue and posterior auricular region.

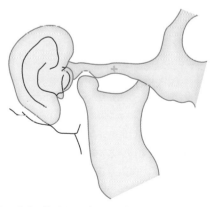

**Fig. 8.3:** Extraoral mandibular nerve block

## *Technique*

The midpoint of the notch between condyle and coronoid process of mandible is palpated under the zygomatic arch. A skin wheal is raised there. A long (about 8 cm) needle is inserted perpendicular to skin until it touches the bone, the pterygoid plate at about 4 cm deep. This is little withdrawn and reinserted a little posteriorly gently to reach the foramen ovale. Paraesthesia may be obtained to the lower teeth and/ or lower lip of the same side. The anaesthetic solution (about 5 ml) may be injected there to block the mandibular nerve.

Care should be taken not to insert the injection needle too deep to enter the pharynx which is a potential infected area.

## *Indications*

1. For extraction of several teeth of the lower jaw
2. For removal of second or third molar tooth.

- For extraction of teeth of the lower jaw a single injection may be enough to make one-half of the lower jaw and tongue painless. The central incisior gets some innervation from the other side. The lateral buccal fold, molar buccal alveolar fold and gum get nerve supply from buccinator nerve. These can be locally infiltrated.

One should locate by palpating the anterior border of the ramus of the mandible, the retromolar fossa and the internal oblique ridge on the particular side, while the mouth is open. The injection needle is introduced along the medial side of this ridge for about 2.5 cm. The syringe is kept parallel to the occlusion plane of lower teeth and the barrel of the syringe will be over the premolar teeth of the opposite side. The local anaesthetic solution (2% lignocaine with adrenaline 2-3 ml) is then injected slowly.

## Lingual Nerve Block

Lingual nerve is a terminal branch of the mandibular nerve. It is the only sensory nerve supplying the floor of mouth between alveolar margin and midline.

The retromolar fossa of the mandible is located and the internal oblique ridge is palpated. A needle is introduced through the buccal mucosa just medial to internal oblique line and 2% lignocaine 2 ml is injected.

### *Indications*

1. Surgery of the tongue
2. Management of malignant pain

The block is often combined with glossopharyngeal nerve block.

## Block of Supraorbital Branches of Ophthalmic Division of Trigeminal Nerve (Figs 8.4 and 8.5)

The nerve is blocked above the eyebrow palpating the supraorbital notch. The nerve emerges on the face through the foramen that lie in the same vertical plane as the pupil when the patient looks straight forward. The needle is inserted perpendicular to forehead at the notch and 2 to 3 ml anaesthetic solution is injected.

• Infiltration of local anaesthetic over the medial half of forehead above the eyebrow will block the supraorbital and

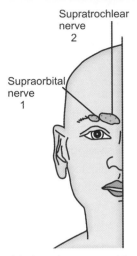

**Fig. 8.4:** Supraorbital and supratrochlear nerve blocks.
1. Supraorbital nerve block; 2. Supratrochlear nerve block

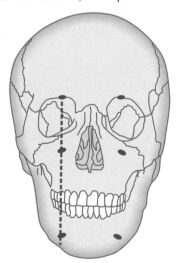

**Fig. 8.5:** Foramina for exit of supraorbital, infraorbital and mental nerves are in one vertical line plane

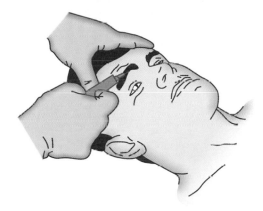

**Fig. 8.6:** Supratrochlear nerve block

supratrochlear branches of ophthalmic nerve. Operations limited to this area can be done with this method (Fig. 8.6).

## Block of Infraorbital Branch of Maxillary Nerve

This terminal branch of maxillary nerve can be blocked at 1 cm below the margin of orbit, below the pupil, when the patient looks forward. Infraorbital foramen is in line of supraorbital notch and canine fossa.

A needle is inserted through a wheal below the midpoint of lower orbit usually 1 cm lateral to ala of the nose. Lignocaine 2% 2 ml can be injected there to provide anaesthesia over the cheek and upper lip. The block can also be done intraorally.

## Mental Nerve Block (Fig. 8.7)

Mental nerve is the terminal branch of ophthalmic nerve and it emerges through the mental foramen of the mandible. It

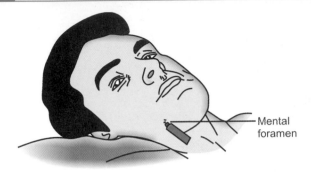

**Fig. 8.7:** Mental nerve block

may vary in position from infancy to old age. The mental foramen is in the same straight vertical plane as the pupil when the patient looks straight forward as is also the second bicuspid tooth. The block can be done either extraorally or intraorally. Analgesia of the lower lip of the same side will result.

## Glossopharyngeal Nerve Block

The glossopharyngeal nerve is the mixed cranial nerve and it leaves the skull through the jugular foramen accompanying internal jugular vein, vagus and accessory nerves. It is enclosed in its own sheath. It passes downwards between the internal carotid artery and the internal jugular vein to the lateral side of vagus.

As it is closely related to vagus and accessory nerves after its exist from skull, it is recommended to block the nerve at a far distal site as it sweeps around the styloid process of temporal bone.

Its sensory supply includes posterior one-third of tongue, pharynx, and superior surface of epiglottis. Its motor supply includes the muscles of deglutition.

## Indications

1. Tic douloureux, glossopharyngeal tic pain
2. Neuralgia of the nerve
3. Cancer pain
4. Anaesthesia in posterior one-third of tongue. It should be combined with lingual nerve block.

## Technique

Patient should lie supine with head turned to opposite side. The mid point of a line joining the tip of mastoid process and the angle of mandible is located. A fine needle is inserted perpendicular to skin until the styloid process is touched at about 3 to 4 cm deep. The needle is little withdrawn and then reinserted further 0.5 cm deep posterior to the styloid process to place the needle point adjacent to the glossopharyngeal nerve.

After proper aspiration test, 3 to 5 ml of the local anaesthetic solution (2% lignocaine) is injected slowly.

Successful block will indicate analgesia of the pharynx, tonsil, soft palate and posterior one-third of the tongue.

## Vagus Nerve Block (Fig. 8.8) (Collins, 1972)

Vagus nerve is a mixed nerve having both motor and sensory functions and a wider distribution than any of the cranial nerves. Its sensory branches to the larynx and trachea are used for regional anaesthesia for intubation procedures and treatment of chronic cancer pain in larynx and/or trachea.

Nerve supply of the larynx and trachea is from vagus through its branches, superior laryngeal nerve and recurrent laryngeal nerve. The superior laryngeal nerve arises near the base of skull

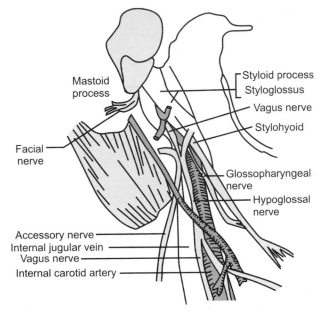

**Fig. 8.8:** Anatomy of vagus and glossopharyngeal nerves

and divides into the internal laryngeal nerve and external laryngeal nerve slightly below and anterior to the greater cornu of the hyoid bone. Internal laryngeal nerve is the sensory nerve of the larynx down to the level of vocal cords. The external laryngeal nerve passes down external to larynx to provide motor supply to cricothyroid muscle and inferior constrictor muscle of the pharynx.

Recurrent laryngeal nerve on the right side of neck passes around the subclavian artery and goes upto the larynx between trachea and oesophagus. But on the left side it arises from vagus in the thorax and loops around the aortic arch and passes to the larynx in the groove between oesophagus and trachea. Recurrent laryngeal nerve supplies all the muscles of the larynx except cricothyroid. It is sensory to the larynx below the vocal cord and to the trachea.

Vagus nerve can be blocked at its exit from the skull at jugular foramen where it lies anteromedial to the internal jugular vein. Cervical sympathetic ganglion and glossopharyngeal, accessory and hypoglossal nerves are closely related to it.

## *Technique*

A skin wheal is raised on the midpoint of the line joining the tip of mastoid process and the angle of mandible. A needle is introduced gently for about 2.5 cm perpendicular to skin. If the styloid process is touched, it may be redirected posteriorly for about 1 cm deeper. The local anaesthetic solution is deposited there after confirmed by aspiration test.

Successful bilateral vagus block will result aphonia, abolition of cough reflex, tachycardia, hypertension and motionless vocal cords. Block of cervical sympathetic may cause Horner's syndrome. Block of hypoglossal nerve may cause fall back of tongue. Glossopharyngeal block may indicate dysphagia.

## Superior Laryngeal Nerve Block (Collins, 1972) (Figs 8.9 and 8.10)

The nerve is blocked at a point above its entrance into larynx through thyrohyoid membrane, slightly below and anterior to greater cornu of hyoid bone. The block may be helpful in cases of laryngectomy, laryngitis, cancer larynx, etc.

The greater cornu of hyoid bone is first identified and located by the finger tip. A skin wheal is formed into the notch of

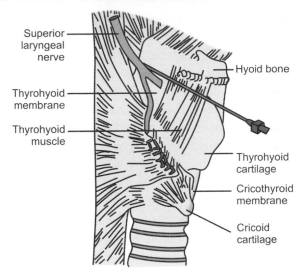

**Fig. 8.9:** Laryngeal nerve block

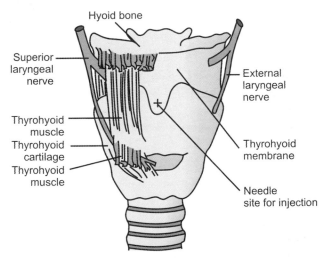

**Fig. 8.10:** Superior laryngeal nerve block

thyroid cartilage in the midline. The needle is then inserted through the wheal and advanced gently to a point just under cornua of hyoid bone. A further deep advancement may injure the vessels of the neck. After proper aspiration test, the anaesthetic solution should be injected slowly. Block of the other side can also be done through the same wheal.

Successful block causes analgesia of the larynx above the cord and the functions like deglutition, phonation, cough, expectoration will suffer.

## Stellate Ganglion Block

The cervical sympathetic chain includes superior, middle and inferior cervical ganglia. The inferior cervical ganglion and first thoracic ganglion usually fuse to form the stellate ganglion. The postganglionic sympathetic supply to the face, upper chest, thoracic viscera, head and arm traverses the stellate ganglion.

The stellate ganglion lies between the transverse process of $C_7$ vertebra and the neck of the first rib, usually on the anterolateral surface of body of $C_7$ vertebra. It is just behind the subclavian artery and origin of vertebral artery. On the right side, the apex of lung and the pleural dome lie anteriorly, but on the left side, these are about 1 cm lower so that the risk of puncture is relatively less.

### *Effects of Stellate Ganglion Block*

1. Horner syndrome (ptosis, miosis, enophthalmos)
2. Vasodilatation in head, neck, face, arm and hand
3. Increased skin temperature
4. Fall in intraocular tension
5. Anhydrosis, inhibition of sweating
6. Inhibition of salivary and bronchial glands

7. Nasal congestion, flushing of cheek, face, neck and arm
8. Inhibition of cardiac pain
9. Inhibition of causalgic pain from upper limb.

## Indications

1. Diagnosis and treatment of reflex sympathetic dystrophies
2. Management of circulatory inadequacy in the upper limb
3. Thrombosis, embolism and spasm of the vessels of head, neck and arm
4. Causalgia of upper limb
5. Anginal pain
6. Pulmonary embolism.

## Technique

The patient should lie supine, chin forwards and the head extended over a pillow and the face turned towards the opposite side. The important landmark for the block is the cricoid cartilage which overlies the $C_6$ vertebra. The transverse process of $C_6$ vertebra (the Chaussignac's tubercle) is most prominent. The block can be done either at the level of $C_6$ or $C_7$ which is about 1 to 2 cm caudal to it. A skin wheal is made 2 cm lateral to jugular notch and 2 cm above the clavicle which is immediately on the medial border of the sternomastoid muscle. The anterior tubercle of $C_7$ vertebra is found by retracting the sternomastoid muscle with the anaesthetist's left hand at this level. It helps to move the carotid artery and internal jugular vein inside the deep cervical fascia out of the way of the needle path.

The 6 cm needle is inserted through the wheal paratracheally between the cricoid cartilage and the laterally retracted sternomastoid muscle. It is advanced directly backwards until it touches the transverse process of the vertebra $C_7$. The needle should be withdrawn a little (0.5 to 1 cm), out of the prevertebral muscles anterior to the prevertebral fascia and then 10 to 15 ml local anaesthetic solution is deposited. Before that, aspiration test for blood or CSF must be done. A test dose of local anaesthetic may also be given to identify the proper space to block the ganglion.

## Complications

1. Pneumothorax, pleural shock
2. Intravascular injection: intravenous or vertebral artery or carotid artery injection. Local anaesthetic systemic toxicity.
3. Subarachnoid injection
4. Recurrent laryngeal nerve block
5. Phrenic nerve block
6. Brachial plexus block
7. Haematoma
8. Block of cardioaccelerator fibres: hypotension, bradycardia
9. Perforation of oesophagus, infection

## Cervical Plexus Block

The cervical plexus is formed by the upper four cervical nerves ($C_1$, $C_2$, $C_3$ and $C_4$ spinal nerves). The cervical plexus supplies skin and muscles of neck and the diaphragm.

Each cervical nerve divides into two, except the first $C_1$. The $C_1$ joins the upper branch of $C_2$, the adjoining upper and lower branches fuse and the lower branch $C_4$ fuses with $C_5$ to form brachial plexus. Thus, three loops are formed and the first loop is directed forwards while the other two are directed backwards.

Cervical plexus is formed anterior to the scalenus medius muscle and deep to sternomastoid muscle and internal jugular vein. The plexus gives rise to superficial (cutaneous) and deep (muscular) branches. The superficial plexus supplies the posterior structures of the neck and head and the upper part of thorax and shoulders. The deep plexus forms in the paravertebral region of $C_2$ $C_3$ and $C_4$ vertebrae and supplies the deep structures of the lateral and anterior region of the neck and gives branches to the phrenic nerve. The deep branches are mostly motor excepting the phrenic nerve which has efferent visceral sensory fibres.

## Indications of Cervical Plexus Block

1. Operations of the neck, thyroidectomy
2. Chronic pain syndromes, cancer pain
3. Neuralgia
4. Deep branches are mostly motor, thus its block has limited indications, more over it may be complicated with vertebral artery injection, phrenic nerve block, subdural or epidural injection and brachial plexus block. The superficial block provides complete sensory block without motor involvement and with less major complications.
5. Tracheostomy.

## Technique of Deep Cervical Plexus Block

Patient should be kept supine with head turning slightly to opposite side and the chin is perpendicular to spine.

The tip of mastoid process and a point corresponding to anterior border of $C_6$ vertebra which is the most prominent cervical vertebra and easily palpable, are located. A line is drawn between the two. $C_2$ corresponds on the line about a finger breadth from mastoid tip. Transverse processes of $C_3$ $C_4$ and $C_5$ will be 2 cm, 3 cm and 4 cm respectively below the level of $C_2$.

Skin wheals are raised at each $C_2$, $C_3$ and $C_4$ level. Three needles are inserted at these skin wheals parpendicular to sagittal plane to touch the bony points at tips of transverse processes of cervical vertebrae. Aspiration test should be done for blood or CSF. The anaesthetic solution is then deposited in each place.

A single needle technique and injection of about 10 ml of anaesthetic solution at the level of $C_4$ may also produce satisfactory block.

### Complications

1. Phrenic nerve block
2. Subarachnoid injection
3. Epidural injection
4. Intravascular injection
5. Vagus block
6. Recurrent laryngeal nerve block
7. Cervical sympathetic block
8. Horner's syndrome.

### Technique of Superficial Cervical Plexus Block

This can be done by injecting about 20 ml of the local anaesthetic solution between skin and muscle at about the midpoint along the posterior border of sternomastoid muscle. It may be used independently or to complement the main deep cervical plexus block.

Successful cervical plexus block provides analgesia on the front and back of neck, occipital region and upper part of thorax and shoulders in a cape-like fashion.

### Phrenic Nerve Block

It can be done at the origin of its roots $C_3$, $C_4$ and $C_5$ near the transverse process of fourth cervical vertebra including $C_3$ and $C_5$ as these usually send contributing branches.

These three nerves can be successfully blocked through the skin wheal at $C_4$. The needle is inserted through the skin wheal to touch the transverse process of $C_4$ vertebra and 5 ml local anaesthetic solution is injected. Then the needle is directed cephalad towards transverse process of $C_3$ and then directed caudal towards transverse process of $C_5$ to block $C_5$.

Diaphragm is innervated by both intercostal nerves and phrenic nerve. Phrenic nerve block usually does not compromise respiration at rest in normal subjects. But it may affect adversely in patients with paraplegia, quadriplegia, spinal cord injury, etc.

## BLOCKS OF THORAX, ABDOMEN AND PERINEUM

### Intercostal Nerve Block (Fig. 8.11)

The intercostal nerves are formed by the anterior primary rami of $T_1$ to $T_{12}$. These are 12 in number on each side. The nerve runs obliquely across the intercostal space to the angle of rib above and is further extended in the subcostal groove accompanied by a thoracic vein and artery. All these are enclosed by the rib above and below and by the external and internal intercostal muscles. This constitutes a space and the local anaesthetic solution is deposited here to block the nerve. The order of the structures is the vein, artery and nerve from above downwards. Intercostal nerve takes the circumferential course around the trunk and supply the intercostal and abdominal muscles and skin on the lateral and anterior walls of the trunk.

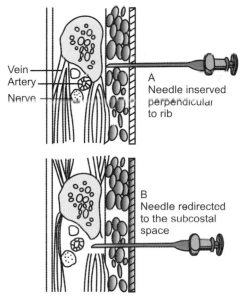

**Fig. 8.11:** Intercostal nerve block

It should be noted that the block of the intercostal nerve beyond the angle of rib is regarded as intercostal block. Block of the thoracic nerves at their exit from the intervertebral foramen is known as paravertebral block which includes posterior divisions and the ramus communicans. Posterior rami supply the skin and the muscles of back.

## Indications of Intercostal Block

1. Pain relief (rib fractures)
2. Postoperative analgesia
3. Anaesthesia for intra-abdominal surgery (Multiple bilateral intercostal block combined with coeliac plexus block).

## Technique of Intercostal Block

Intercostal nerve can be blocked at any accessible point in its course. It may be posterior, lateral or anterior. It is usually done posteriorly at the angle of ribs for surgical anaesthesia.

Patient should lie in prone or lateral position with the shoulder abducted to rotate the scapula superiorly and laterally. Block is better performed lateral to posterior, midline at the angle of rib (about 8-10 cm from the midline) as the ribs are easily palpated and identified and the intercostal space is relatively wide. Moreover, the lateral cutaneous branches are not yet left the intercostal space.

The lower border of the rib is palpated and skin wheal is made over the intercostal space. The skin overlying the rib is drawn upwards and a short bevel 5 cm needle is inserted at a slightly cephalad angle to touch the periosteum of rib. The needle is well supported by fingers and then "walked" off the inferior edge of the rib as the skin which was drawn upwards returns to its normal position. Then the needle is carefully advanced for 3 to 4 mm until it slips under its lower edge and penetrates the external intercostal muscle at its origin in the intercostal groove. A loss of resistance can be felt. Paraesthesia may occur but it is not necessary to elicit.

After aspiration test 5 ml of 1% lignocaine with adrenaline should be injected.

A series of intercostal blocks from $T_4$ to $T_{12}$ will be needed to produce satisfactory analgesic effect on the anterior abdominal wall. For intra-abdominal surgery this should be combined with proper celiac plexus block. For abdominal and chest operations and for rib fractures on anterior parts, intercostal block should be done in midaxillary or postaxillary line. In patients with poor general condition where minimum movement is desirable the block can also be done in supine position. For operations of longer duration, bupivacaine should be used. Otherwise, lignocaine 1 to 1.5% with adrenaline may be quite satisfactory.

## Complications

1. Intravascular injection, systemic toxicity
2. Pneumothorax due to inadvertent puncture of lungs.
3. Bilateral intercostal blocks over a wide area need large volume of local anaesthetic and there is risk of rapid absorption from the vascular intercostal space and systemic toxicity. Indwelling intercostal space catheters may be used for long-term anaesthesia. It avoids the need for repeated injections.

## Intercostal Block for Rib Resection

1. The patient is placed with lateral position with head and shoulders elevated.
2. The line of incision is noted and it is infiltrated with 1% lignocaine solution.
3. An intradermal and subcutaneous line of infiltration should be done one rib above and one rib below the length of rib to be resected.

4. These line of infiltration should well extend at least 3 cm in front and posteriorly. These end points are joined with infiltration.

5. Intercostal nerves within this infiltrated area are blocked at their posterior ends with 2% lignocaine solution.

6. Anaesthesia is mostly satisfactory. But mild discomfort may be there during cutting of the periosteum of the rib.

### Interpleural Block

Continuous interpleural block is indicated for prolonged pain relief following thoracic surgery, in the postoperative period. It may also be used to produce analgesia due to fracture ribs.

Here an epidural (Tuohy) needle filled with saline upto the hub is inserted at the cephalad margin of the 5th, 6th or 7th rib and advanced gently until it pierces the parietal pleura. Here, the saline at the hub is sucked into the pleural cavity. Extreme care is essential not to puncture the visceral pleura. An epidural catheter is then passed through the needle and about 5 to 6 cm of the catheter should lie in the thoracic cavity. The needle is the removed gently over the catheter. The catheter is well secured and a sterile dressing is applied. The patient is placed supine.

Bupivacaine 0.25% or 0.5% solution (20-25 ml) may be injected through the catheter. The block may be continued with repeated injections or an infusion.

### *Complications*

1. Pneumothorax
2. Lung injury
3. Intravascular injection
4. Catheter problems: kinking, misplacement, occlusion, infection, etc.

## Abdominal Field Block (Fig. 8.12) (Collins, 1972)

The abdominal wall is innervated by the lower six thoracic nerves. At the anterior end of the intercostal space, the nerves pass behind the costal cartilages and run forwards between the internal oblique and the transversus abdominis before they pierce the lateral margin of rectus sheath. The terminals pierce the muscle and supply it and supply the skin of the anterior abdominal wall.

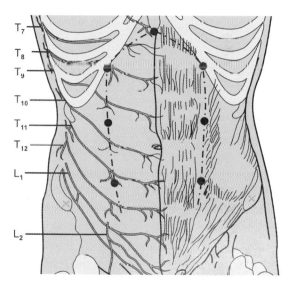

**Fig. 8.12:** Abdominal field block

### *Sensory Nerve Supply of Abdominal Wall*

1. The region of nipple: $T_5$
2. Epigastrium: $T_7$
3. Umbilicus: $T_{10}$

4. Midway between umbilicus and pubis: $T_{12}$
5. Groin: $L_1$

### Important Landmarks

1. Xiphoid on a level of body of $T_9$
2. Subcostal plane at $L_3$
3. Highest point of iliac crest at $L_4$

### Indications of Abdominal Field Block

1. Abdominal wall surgery
2. Painful scars in abdominal wall
3. Intra-abdominal surgery can be done with abdominal field block in combination with coeliac plexus block. Only abdominal field block provides the abdominal wall and its underlying parietal peritonium insensitive.

### Technique

The block may be done either in axillary line or in nipple line. If axillary line is used, infiltration should be done into the deep fasia, but in nipple line it should be inside the muscle sheath.

Skin wheals are done in several points: (a) one at the tip of xiphoid process ($T_9$), (b) bilaterally at the costal margin of the 9th rib where rectus muscles cross it, (c) one on each side of lateral margin of the rectus just above the umbilicus, and (d) one on each side of the lateral margin of rectus below umbilicus.

Through each of the lateral wheals, the needle is inserted towards the rectus sheath to pierce the muscle and the anaesthetic solution is deposited there. Then further anaesthetic solution is injected subcutaneously so as to join the skin wheals. Similarly the skin wheal at the tip of xiphoid precess is also joined to the wheals along the costal margin.

A large volume of anaesthetic solution (100 to 200 ml) may be needed.

The block may provide satisfactory analgesia and muscular relaxation, but for extensive intra-abdominal procedure the relaxation may not be adequate.

### Rectus-sheath Block (Fig. 8.13)

Here the needle is directed to pierce the anterior layer of rectus sheath and the anaesthetic solution is placed posterior to the muscle, so that the intercostal nerves are blocked together with the zone of skin medial to its outer border. It produces an excellent muscular relaxation. But care should be taken not to perforate peritonium.

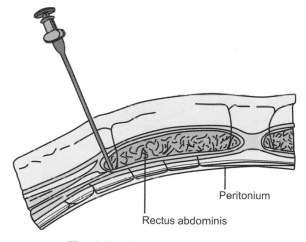

Peritonium

Rectus abdominis

**Fig. 8.13:** Rectus sheath block

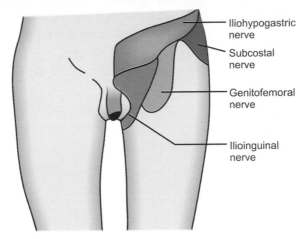

**Fig. 8.14:** Cutaneous nerve supply of groin

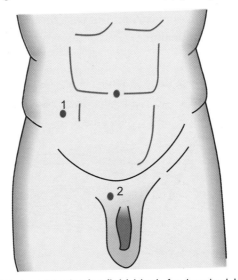

**Fig. 8.15:** Landmarks for field block for inguinal hernia.
1. Anterior superior iliac spine; 2. Pubic tubercle

## Field Block of the Inguinal Region (Figs 8.14 and 8.15)

The inguinal canal is about 1.5 inches long and extends from the internal inguinal ring laterally and external inguinal ring medially and lies above medial half of the inguinal ligament. The internal inguinal ring is an opening in the transversalis fascia just above the midpoint of inguinal ligament. The external inguinal ring is an opening in the external oblique and lies above and lateral to the pubic tubercle.

The inguinal canal contains the ilioinguinal nerve and the spermatic cord in males or the round ligament of the uterus in females. The spermatic cord includes the vas deferens, internal and external spermatic arteries, arteries to vas deferens, pampiniform venous plexus, lymphatic vessels and autonomic nerve fibres.

Inguinal region is innervated from $T_{11}$, $T_{12}$, $L_1$ and $L_2$ nerves through iliohypogastric ($T_{12}$, $L_1$), ilioinguinal ($T_{12}$ $L_1$), subcostal ($T_{12}$) and genitofemoral ($L_1$ and $L_2$) and subcutaneous ramifications of other adjacent nerves. Autonomic nerve fibres from the lower thoracic segments descend with and supply the spermatic cord and its contents.

### Indications

1. Repair of hernia
2. Postoperative pain relief.

### Contraindications

1. Not suitable for children
2. Noncooperative patients
3. Irreducible hernia in obese patient.

*Technique*

Essential landmarks are:

1. Pubic tubercle
2. Anterior superior iliac spine
3. Half inch above the midpoint of inguinal ligament.

A skin wheal is raised about 3 cm internal to anterior superior iliac spine. A long needle is inserted vertically backwards until it pierces the external oblique aponeurosis with a slight click. After aspiration test, the anaesthetic solution (1% lignocaine about 30 ml) is injected to block the ilioinguinal and iliohypogastric nerves. Solution is also deposited in all layers between the wheal and anterior superior iliac spine.

A second wheal is formed over the pubic tubercle and a long needle is inserted for intradermal and subcutaneous injection in the direction of umbilicus to block the overlapping nerves from the opposite side.

A third wheal is formed half inch above the midinguinal ligament and a needle is inserted perpendicularly to pierce the aponeurosis of external oblique. About 20 ml anaesthetic solution is injected to block the genital branch of the genitofemoral nerve. Prior needle insertion, one should confirm that the inguinal canal does not contain hernial contents.

Infiltration along the line of incision may be given for further satisfaction.

Infiltration of local anaesthetic solution round the neck of sac is often helpful to avoid the discomfort during manipulation of the sac.

## Coeliac Plexus Block

The coeliac plexus is the largest plexus of sympathetic system. The plexus lies at the level of $L_1$ vertebra anterior to the lower half of the body of $T_{12}$ and entire body of $L_1$ vertebra. It is in between the adrenal gland and behind the stomach and other viscera. It is in front of crura of the diaphragm. It is extraperitoneal and being surrounded by loose areolar tissues.

It is composed of a dense network of ganglia and nerve fibres around the coeliac artery. The plexus derives nerves from:

1. Sympathetic preganglionic fibres carried through greater splanchnic nerves and lesser splanchnic nerves.
2. Sympathetic postganglionic fibres directly from the upper lumbar ganglia.
3. Parasympathetic fibres from the vagus nerves.

Greater splanchnic nerve is derived 6th, 7th, 8th and 9th thoracic sympathetic ganglion. The lesser splanchnic nerve is derived from 10th and 11th thoracic sympathetic ganglion. The coeliac plexus sends postganglionic sympathetic fibres to the abdominal organs and receives nociceptive transmission from organs like pancreas.

## *Indications of Coeliac Plexus Block*

1. To relieve visceral pain from the distal oesophagus to the descending colon.
2. To relieve cancer pain in upper abdomen
3. Treatment of acute pancreatitis
4. *Intra-abdominal surgery*: often combined with abdominal field block. Regional anaesthesia in such cases requires multiple injections and large volume of local anaesthetic drugs. Thus, it is not in vogue in recent times.
5. Coeliac plexus block with alcohol or phenol is used to treat pancreatic cancer pain.

*Technique*

The patient is placed in a prone position. The skin wheal is performed about 8 cm from the midline at the interior edge of the twelfth rib. Then a 22 gauge long needle is inserted through the wheal and advanced 45° towards the vertebral body. It will touch the lateral body of $L_1$ vertebra at about 10 to 12 cm depth. After contact with the vertebral body the needle is little withdrawn and redirected at a steeper angle so that it will slide off the vertebral body and lie in the periaortic region.

Needle position may be confirmed with the help of radiography or computed tomographic scan. A 2 ml test dose of the local anaesthetic solution may be given to note the results. Aspiration test for blood should also be done. The anaesthetic solution of about 25 ml may be given gently. The similar block should also be done on the other side in the usual manner.

*Complications*

1. Hypotension
2. Increased gastric motility
3. Retroperitoneal haematoma
4. Intravascular injection
5. Kidney puncture
6. Block of somatic nerves
7. Systemic local anaesthetic toxicity.

**Paravertebral Nerve Blocks**

Paravertebral segmental nerves can be blocked in the paravertebral space which is a wedge shaped compartment close to the vertebral column where the nerve trunks emerge from the intervertebral foramina. One paravertebral space has no direct communication with another, but may communicate indirectly through the intervertebral foramina with extradural space. Thus, local anaesthetic spread from one paravertebral space to another can occur across the extradural space and block the adjacent nerves on the same or the opposite side of the body. The nerves can be blocked in the paravertebral space from $C_1$ to $L_5$. When $T_1$ to $L_2$ nerve roots are blocked, their rami communicantes are also blocked.

Paravertebral blocks either thoracic or lumbar can be done in either the prone or lateral position. The technique is mostly similar. Firstly, the transverse process or the lamina of the proper vertebra should be located and identified. Then the needle should be walked off the transverse process or lamina to enter into the paravertebral space where the injection is to be made.

Common *indications* are for diagnosis and treatment of chronic pain syndromes. It is more indicated where the spinal or epidural blocks are not feasible or otherwise contraindicated.

### Paravertebral Thoracic Block

The spinous processes of the thoracic vertebrae are rounded and increase in length and slope from above downward so that in the midthoracic region the spine may overlap the vertebral level two spinal segments below. The tip of 4th to 9th spinous process is either on a level of the next rib or next lower intercostal space.

### Technique (Pinnock et al)

The appropriate spinous process of the vertebra is located. A skin wheal is performed 4 to 5 cm lateral to spinous process.

A long 10 cm needle is inserted directly perpendicular to skin until it touches the lateral transverse process at a depth of 3 to 5 cm. The needle is then partially withdrawn and reinserted upwards until it glances off the cephalad edge of transverse process. Then it is advanced gently for about 2 cm to pass through costotransverse ligament. A change in tissue resistance can be felt when it enters the loose fatty paravertebral space.

Loss of resistance to saline can be used to confirm the location of needle point. Aspiration test for blood and CSF should always be done to avoid vascular puncture or dural puncture. Then the anaesthetic solution 5 ml 1.5% lignocaine can be deposited.

It should be noted a single injection may affect 1 to 6 dermatomes and can produce bilateral block due to spread through epidural space. For extensive block, the procedure can be repeated in another suitable space or a catheter may be introduced to give incremental doses of local anaesthetic.

### *Complications*

1. Pneumothorax
2. Subarachnoid injection
3. Vascular injection, systemic toxicity
4. Extensive epidural spread.

### Paravertebral Lumbar Block

In the lumbar region the spinous processes are long and wide and the transverse processes are short. The upper edge of the spinous process of a lumbar vertebra is mostly at the level with the transverse process of that vertebra.

A skin wheal is raised opposite the upper end of the spine of the vertebra, about 4 cm lateral to the midline. A long

10 cm needle is inserted through the wheal at right angle to skin and advanced to contact transverse process at a depth of about 4 to 5 cm. Then the needle is little withdrawn and directed slightly upwards and inwards so that it is walked posteriorly off the transverse process. The needle is further advanced 1 to 2 cm to enter in the paravertebral space. The anaesthetic solution (1.5% lignocaine 5 ml) is gently deposited thereafter aspiration test for blood or CSF.

*Successful paravertebral block* from $T_1$ to $L_2$ provides visceral block along with the analgesic effect on the abdominal wall due to the block of the white rami as well.

Paravertebral somatic block can provide regional anaesthesia in various operations such as appendicectomy ($T_{10}$–$L_2$), repair of hernia ($T_{11}$ to $L_2$), upper abdominal operations ($T_5$ to $T_{12}$), lower abdominal operations ($T_7$ to $L_3$). But these blocks are not used nowadays.

### Thoraco-lumbar Sympathetic Block

The location of the sympathetic chain and ganglia is on the anterolateral surface of bodies of vertebra. They lie anterior to the somatic nerves.

The patient should lie either in prone or in lateral position. The spinous processes of the appropriate vertebrae are identified. In the thoracic region a skin wheal is performed 4 to 5 cm lateral to the tip of the spine. In the lumbar region it is done at the upper border of the spine. A long needle is inserted through the wheal perpendicular to skin and advanced to touch the bone either rib or transverse process. Then the needle is slightly withdrawn and redirected downwards at about 30° for thoracic ganglia and upwards for lumbar ganglia. The body of vertebra is contacted and the needle is just slided off. The local anaesthetic solution (1.5% lignocaine 5 ml) is then gently deposited to block.

Continuous catheter technique can also be performed for sympathetic block.

### Indications

1. Causalgias
2. Thrombophlebitis
3. Herpes zoster
4. Cancer pain
5. Phantom limb

### Complications

1. Neuritis, neuralgia
2. Subarachnoid injection

### Penile Block

The sensory nerve supply of penis is from the terminal branches of the internal pudendal nerves, the dorsal nerves of penis. The skin at the base of penis is supplied by ilioinguinal and genitofemoral nerves.

The patient should be placed supine. The distal edge of the symphysis pubis is located. A needle is inserted in the midline at the base of penis and advanced off the symphysis pubis at which point it should have passed through the deep Buck's fasia of penis. Then the local anaesthetic solution 5 to 7 ml is injected after careful negative aspiration test for blood. Vasoconstrictor like adrenaline should never be used in the local anaesthetic as arteries of the penis are end arteries.

Both the dorsal nerves of penis are mostly blocked with this technique. The block should then be completed by subcutaneous ring infiltration across the root of penis. The infiltration should be started 2 cm lateral to midline and continuously advanced across the median raphe and ends about 2 cm beyond it on the other side. Urethra is very superficial at the base of penis, so the injection should be strictly subcutaneous.

The block is indicated for circumcision and for postoperative pain relief after repair of hypospadius.

## Perineal Anaesthesia

The perineum is mainly innervated by the internal pudendal nerve with its three branchs such as the dorsal nerve of penis or clitoris, the labial or scrotal nerve and the inferior haemorrhoidal nerve. The pudendal nerve is the largest nerve of the pudendal plexus. It is derived from $S_2$, $S_3$ and $S_4$ nerves. It leaves the pelvic cavity through the lower part of greater sciatic foramen and then passes behind the ischial spine lying posteror to sacrospinous ligament and then through the lesser sciatic foramen to enter the perineum. Thus, the nerve can be easily blocked just medial and posterior to the ischial tuberosity by infiltration of local anaesthetic solution. It gives the main sensory supply to the perineum, vulva and lower two-third of vagina. The other sensory supply to the vulva includes ilioinguinal nerve and perineal branches of the posterior cutaneous nerve of the thigh.

## Pudendal Nerve Block

### Indications

1. To provide perineal analgesia for low outlet forceps delivery.
2. For simple haemorrhoid operations.

### Technique

#### Transvaginal approach

The patient is placed in lithotomy position with careful antiseptic precautions. The ischial spine is located by index finger inserted vaginally. The sacrospinous ligament can be easily palpated. A long needle is inserted lateral to the finger through the vaginal wall behind the ischial spine. The needle is advanced to pierce the tough sacrospinous ligament and then a loss of resistance can be felt. The needle is kept in position and aspiration test for blood is done. Following negative aspiration, about 8 to 10 ml of the anaesthetic solution is deposited to block the pudendal nerve at this point. The procedure should be repeated on the other side.

#### Transperineal approach (Fig. 8.16)

The patient is in lithotomy position. The posteromedial margin of the ischial tuberosity is palpated over the perineum. A skin wheal is raised at midpoint of line joining anus and the ischial tuberosity. A long needle is inserted through the wheal and advanced to the ischial spine which is palpated by a finger in vagina. The needle is further advanced to reach behind the ischial spine. After negative aspiration test, 8 to 10 ml of the local anaesthetic solution are injected. Similar block should also be done on the other side.

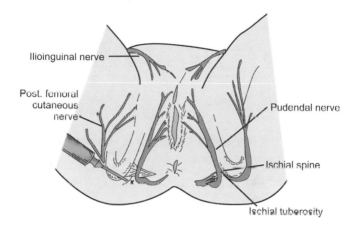

**Fig. 8.16:** Innervation of female perineum and transperineal pudendal nerve block

*Complications*

1. Failure of the block
2. Intravascular injection
3. Systemic toxicity

*Contraindications*

1. Patient sensitivity to local anaesthetics
2. Patient refusal.

## BLOCKS OF UPPER LIMB

### Brachial Plexus Block (Fig. 8.17)

Brachial plexus is formed by the anterior primary rami of $C_5$, $C_6$, $C_7$, $C_8$ and $T_1$ with communications with from $C_4$ and $T_2$. It consists of roots, trunks, divisions, cords and branches.

The roots and trunks are in the neck, the divisions behind the clavicle and the cords and branches lie in the axilla. It should be noted that the subclavian artery is related to roots and trunks and the axillary artery to cords and branches.

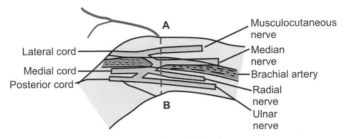

**Fig. 8.17:** Brachial plexus

$C_5$ and $C_6$ roots join to from the upper trunk, $C_7$ alone form the middle trunk and $C_8$ and $T_1$ join to form the lower trunk. All the trunks divide into anterior and posterior division. All the posterior divisions join together to form the posterior cord. The upper two anterior divisions join to form the lateral cord while the lowest anterior division alone forms the medial cord.

Major branches from the cords are as follows:

1. *From medial cord:*
   - Medial head of median $C_8$, $T_1$
   - Medial anterior thoracic $C_8$, $T_1$
   - Ulnar nerve $C_8$, $T_1$
   - Medial cutaneous of forearm $C_8$, $T_1$
   - Medial cutaneous of arm $T_1$
2. *From lateral cord:*
   - Lateral anterior thoracic $C_5$, $C_6$, $C_7$
   - Lateral head of median $C_5$, $C_6$, $C_7$
   - Musculocutaneous $C_5$, $C_6$, $C_7$

*3. From posterior cord:*

- Radial $C_5$, $C_6$, $C_7$, $C_8$, $T_1$
- Axillary $C_5$, $C_6$
- Thoracodorsal $C_6$, $C_7$ $C_8$
- Subscapular $C_5$, $C_6$

The brachial plexus is mostly ensheathed by an extension of the prevertebral fascia from the cervical vertebrae. The presence of this fibrous envelope up to several centimetres distal to axilla helps to block brachial plexus at several sites depending upon the situation.

The scalenus anterior muscle originates from anterior tubercle of transverse processes of $C_3$, $C_4$, $C_5$, and $C_6$ and inserts into the scalene tubercle of the first rib. It separates the subclavian vein from subclavian artery which is posterior to this insertion. The middle scalenus muscle arises from posterior tubercle of transverse process of the lower $C_6$ vertebra and its insertion is separated from scalenus anterior muscle by the groove for subclavian artery.

The roots of brachial plexus run between anterior and posterior tubercles of transverse processes of cervical vertebrae towards the first rib in the interscalene space. As the roots travel down through the space, they join to form the trunks of plexus. Along with subclavian artery these are ensheathed to form the subclavian perivascular sheath which becomes the axillary sheath below the clavicle.

Musculocutaneous nerve arises high in axilla and the axillary nerve leaves the neuro-vascular bundle at the level of pectoralis muscle and thus these nerves may be missed with an axillary approach of brachial plexus block.

## Supraclavicular Brachial Plexus Block
## (Longnecker and Murphy, 1997) (Fig. 8.18)

The block is performed in subclavian perivascular sheath at the site where the plexus crosses the first rib.

The patient should lie supine with a small pillow under the head and neck turning the head slightly away on the opposite side. A point is located 1 cm above and just lateral to the midclavicular point. A skin wheal is made. The subclavian artery is palpated.

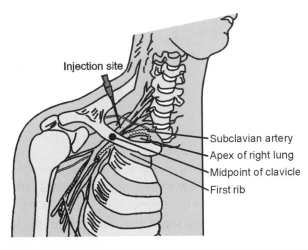

Injection site

Subclavian artery
Apex of right lung
Midpoint of clavicle
First rib

**Fig. 8.18:** Brachial plexus block (supraclavicular approach)

A fine needle of about 5 cm length in inserted through the wheal immediately posterior to subclavian artery inclined at 80° to the skin and directed backwards, inwards and downwards to contact the first rib. Paraesthesia may occur to indicate the contact with the plexus. When there is no paraesthesia, the needle is little walked off the inferior margin of the rib. About 20 ml of 1.5% lignocaine with adrenaline (1 in 200000) is injected in the intercostal space after negative aspiration test for blood. If the subclavian artery is punctured the needle should be withdrawn little a few millimetres outside the artery, then injection can be made while the needle point is still within the sheath.

### Complications

1. Pneumothorax
2. Block of phrenic nerve
3. Block of recurrent laryngeal nerve
4. Block of vagus nerve
5. Block of sympathetic nerves, Horner's syndrome
6. Intravascular injection
7. Systemic texicity of local anaesthetics
8. Risk of subarachnoid / epidural block

### Axillary Block of Brachial Plexus (Fig. 8.19)

The axillary approach is usually indicated for operative procedures distal to elbow and particularly for hand surgery. Here, the musculocutaneous nerve is not usually blocked as it leaves the sheath proximal to the injection point.

The patient should lie supine, the arm is abducted to 90° and externally rotated. The axillary artery is palpated and traced as high as possible to axilla. A needle is inserted just above the artery directed cephalad into the axillary sheath. A definite popping sensation may be felt as the sheath is penetrated. The needle will pulsate with arterial pulsations.

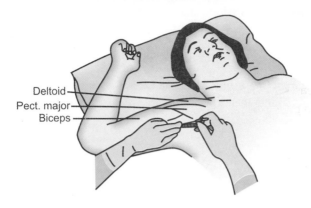

Deltoid
Pect. major
Biceps

**Fig. 8.19:** Brachial plexus block (Axillary approach)

Paraesthesia may occur, but it is not mandatory to elicit paraesthesia to confirm the correct needle placement. A suitable nerve stimulator may be used to confirm the location.

Aspiration test for blood is needed to avoid intravascular injection. After negative aspiration test, the local anaesthetic solution 25 to 30 ml is injected within the sheath. Digital pressure may be applied distal to the needle during and after injection to encourage the spread of the anaesthetic solution within the sheath towards the site where the musculocutaneous nerve exits.

Separate direct block of the musculocutaneous nerve can also be performed. Lignocaine 1.5% with adrenaline is mostly used. But bupivacaine 0.25 to 0.5% can also be used.

Following injection the arm should be adducted and the axilla massaged to promote the anaesthetic spread.

## Advantages

1. No risk of phrenic nerve block, vagus block, recurrent laryngeal nerve block and stellate ganglion block
2. No risk of subarachnoid or epidural block
3. Least risk of pneumothorax
4. No paraesthesia needed.

## Disadvantages

1. Large volumes of anaesthetic solution is needed.
2. Intravascular injection
3. Systemic toxicity
4. It may be difficult in obese patients
5. It cannot be done where the arm cannot be abducted
6. Surgery of the shoulder and upper arm is not possible.

### Interscalene Block

Brachial plexus can also be blocked into the interscalene groove opposite the transverse process of $C_6$ vertebra. The external jugular vein may sometimes overlie this site. In this technique the cephalad roots of brachial plexus are blocked to involve the anterior shoulder, lateral elbow and forearm. Here $C_8$ and $T_1$ are mostly spared and thus the technique is not suitable for surgery on the ulnar aspect of hand and forearm.

The patient should lie supine with head turned to opposite side and a roll placed between the shoulders. The patient's hand is placed on the thigh so as to depress the clavicle. At the level of cricoid cartilage, the posterior border of clavicular head of sternomastoid muscle is located. It is at the level of transverse process of $C_6$ verterbra. Just behind and deep to this, the interscalene groove (between anterior and middle scalene muscles) is identified. Asking the patient to inspire vigorously or shift may help to locate the position of the groove better.

The needle is inserted at this point at right angle to skin and the direction should be caudal, posterior and medial. The needle is advanced further. Paraesthesia may be elicited or the needle may touch the transverse process of cervical vertebrae. Aspiration test for blood should be done before injection. Twenty to 30 ml of local anaesthetic solution should be deposited. A larger volume may spread cephalad to block $C_2$, $C_3$ and $C_4$ nerve roots to produce anaesthesia of cervical plexus.

### Advantages

1. The technique is mostly easy
2. Suitable for shoulder manipulations
3. No risk of pneumothorax.

### Disadvantages

1. Absence of ulnar nerve block
2. Subarachnoid/epidural block can occur
3. Intravascular injection, systemic toxicity
4. Phrenic nerve block can occur
5. Laryngeal nerve block can occur
6. Horner's syndrome.

## Suprascapular Nerve Block (Fig. 8.20)

The nerve arises from $C_5$ and $C_6$ spinal nerves, the upper trunk of brachial plexus. It supplies the shoulder joint, the acromio-clavicular joint, the supraspinatus and infraspinatus muscles. It is the main pathway of somatic pain of these joints and the structures surrounding them. Its block does not provide any skin analgesia.

The nerve may be blockd at the suprascapular notch by approaching posteriorly.

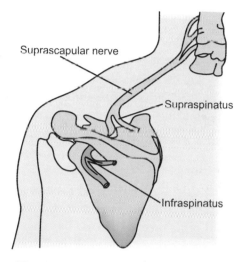

**Fig. 8.20:** Suprascapular nerve block

*Indications*

Shoulder pain due to fibrosities, capsular tears, subacromial bursitis, painful abduction of the arm, calcified shoulder joint. The block is not used for surgery.

*Technique*

The patient should be sitting with arms to his sides and head and shoulder should be slightly flexed.

The spine of the scapula is palpated and its midpoint is identified. The suprascapular notch is about 1 cm above the midpoint. A skin wheal is made there. A short bevel 22 G needle is inserted through the wheal at right angle to the skin. The needle is advanced 2 to 3 cm deep downwards and medially, to contact the bony surface of the supraspinatus fossa, just lateral to notch.

The needle is then carefully withdrawn a little and reintroduced more medially to reach the suprascapular notch. Paraesthesia may be felt at the tip of shoulder. After negative aspiration, 10 ml of the local anaesthetic solution is injected. A nerve stimulator may help to locate the exact site. The needle should not enter into the notch, otherwise nerve damage may occur.

### Ulnar Nerve Block

The ulnar nerve is derived from $C_8$ and $T_1$ nerve roots. $C_8$ and $T_1$ fibres combine to form the lower trunk, most of which becomes the medial cord of the brachial plexus. The ulnar nerve arises from the medial cord and descends on the medial side of the arm. It passes in the ulnar groove at the elbow where it is easily palpable. Then it enters the forearm and descends to wrist where it lies between the ulnar artery and flexor carpi ulnaris tendon. It passes superficial to the transverse carpal ligament into the palm lying medial to the ulnar artery (Fig. 8.21).

The ulnar nerve gives motor supply to the muscles of ulnar side of forearm and most of the short muscles of hand and sensory distribution to the skin and bone of the same area.

### Ulnar Nerve Block at Elbow (Fig. 8.22)

Patient should lie supine, arm abducted to 90° at the shoulder, forearm supinated and elbow flexed to 90°. The medial

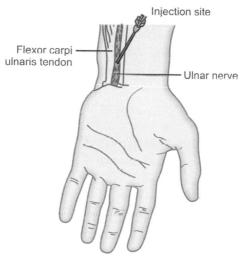

**Fig. 8.21:** Ulnar nerve block at wrist

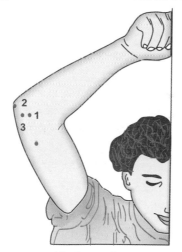

**Fig. 8.22:** Ulnar nerve block at elbow. 1. Medial epicondyle of humerus; 2. Olecranon; 3. Site for injection

epicondyle of humerus is palpated. The ulnar nerve can be palpated in the groove between medial epicondyle of the humerus and olecranon.

A skin wheal is raised over the palpated nerve and near the lower edge of the groove. A fine needle is inserted through the wheal and advanced upwards in groove for about 0.5 to 1cm. Paraesthesia may be elicited if the needle touches the nerve. If the needle touches the bone, it should be repositioned. After negative aspiration test, 3 to 4 ml of local anaesthetic solution is deposited.

### *Ulnar Nerve Block at Wrist (Fig. 8.23)*

The arm is kept supine and the structures like flexor carpi ulnaris tendon, ulnar artery pulse and piseform bone are identified at the skin crease of the wrist. Here, the ulnar nerve lies medial

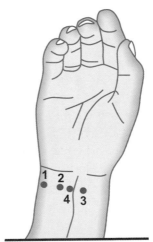

**Fig. 8.23:** Ulnar nerve block at wrist. 1. Styloid process of ulna; 2. Ulnaris tendon; 3. Palmaris longus tendon; 4. Site for injection

to the ulnar artery and deep to the radial border of flexor carpi ulnaris tendon.

A skin wheal is raised between the tendon and artery pulsation. A short needle is inserted perpendicular to skin. Paraesthesia may be obtained. If there is no paraesthesia, the needle may be redirected a little behind the tendon. After negative aspiration test for blood, about 5 ml of the local anaesthetic solution is injected gently.

## Median Nerve Block

The median nerve is derived from $C_6$, $C_7$, $C_8$ and $T_1$ spinal nerves. It originates in two roots arising from the medial and lateral cords of the brachial plexus. The nerve descends first along the lateral side of the brachial artery, then crosses it anteriorly to run on the medial side into the cubital fossa just proximal to the flexor skin crease. Here it is just deep to the bicipital aponeurosis in groove between biceps tendon and origin of forearm flexor muscles.

The median nerve enters the hand deep to the flexor retinaculum in the carpal tunnel.

The median nerve supplies all the muscles on the front of forearm (except flexor carpi ulnaris and ulnar part of flexor digitorum profundus) and in the palm it supplies the short muscle of thumb (except the adductor) and the lateral two lumbricals. The sensory distribution includes the radial side of the palm.

### *Median Nerve block at Elbow (Fig. 8.24)*

The patient should lie supine, the arm abducted at 45°. Then it is held in extension. The brachial artey is palpated between the biceps tendon and the head of pronator teres just proximal to the flexor skin crease of the antecubital fossa.

A short bevel needle is inserted just medial to the brachial artery and 1 to 2 cm proximal to flexor skin crease. There may be a pop or loss of resistance as the needle pierces the bicipital aponeurosis. After negative aspiration test, 3 to 5 ml of local anaesthetic solution is injected gently. Paraesthesia may be obtained, if the needle touches the nerve.

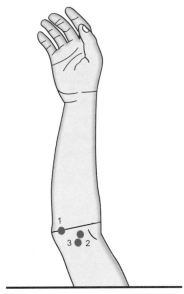

**Fig. 8.24:** Median nerve block at elbow. 1. Intercondylar line; 2. Brachial artery; 3. Site for injection

*Median Nerve Block at Wrist (Fig. 8.25)*

At the wrist the median nerve lies behind the deep fascia of the forearm between the tendons of palmaris longus and flexor carpi radialis. These tendons become more prominent when the patient is asked to flex the wrist while the fist is closed or the flexion is opposed (Fig. 8.26).

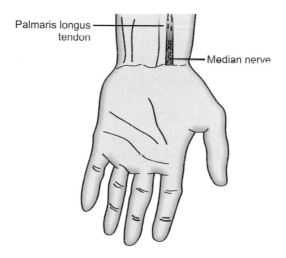

Palmaris longus tendon

Median nerve

**Fig. 8.25:** Median nerve at wrist

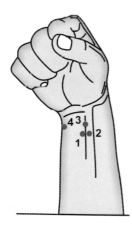

**Fig. 8.26:** Median nerve block at wrist. 1. Palmaris longus tendon; 2. Flexor carpi radialis tendon; 3. Site for injection; 4. Styloid process of ulna

A skin wheal is raised between the tendons of flexor carpi ulnaris and pulmaris longus on the wrist line. A needle is passed through the wheal perpendicular to skin. It is advanced further to pierce the deep fascia of the forearm. Then the 3 to 5 ml of local anaesthetic solution can be gently injected after aspiration test. Paraesthesia to the radial side of palm may be obtained.

## Radial Nerve Block

The radial nerve is derived from $C_5$, $C_6$, $C_7$, $C_8$ and $T_1$ spinal nerves. It originates through the three trunks and the posterior divisions of the trunks to form the posterior cord. The direct continuation of the posterior cord of the brachial plexus is radial nerve. It descends with the axillary artery and brachial artery.

It is the largest branch of brachial plexus. It supplies the extensor muscles of the upper arm and the skin overlying them. It also supplies the extensor muscles of forearm and terminates in its cutaneous nerves to the hand. These digital branches supply the dorsal aspects of the thumb, index and adjacent side of middle finger. The lateral side of middle finger is supplied either by ulnar, radial or both nerves.

The posterior cutaneous nerve of the forearm is the branch of radial nerve. It runs along the posterolateral aspect of forearm to innervate the overlying skin.

### *Radial Nerve Block at Elbow (Fig. 8.27)*

The arm should be positioned with the elbow extended. The intermuscular groove between biceps and brachioradialis muscle at the flexion crease at elbow is located. The nerve usually runs deep to the brachioradialis muscle at this site.

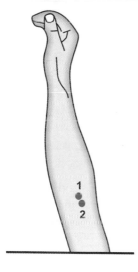

**Fig. 8.27:** Radial nerve block at elbow. 1. Cleft between brachioradialis muscle and biceps tendon; 2. Site for injection

The lateral epicondyle is identified and a finger should be placed to guide the needle direction.

A skin wheal is raised about 2 cm lateral to biceps tendon at the level of flexion crease. A needle is inserted perpendicular to skin into the intermuscular groove and directed towards the lateral epicondyle. Paraesthesia may be obtained. Use of a nerve stimulator may help to locate the nerve position. After negative aspiration test for blood, 5 to 8 ml of local anaesthetic solution may be deposited to block the radial nerve.

### Radial Nerve Block at the Wrist

At the wrist the radial nerve diverges the radial artery laterally and posteriorly and pierces the deep fascia.

The arm should be prone and abducted from the body. Anatomical snuff box is identified by extending the thumb under resistance. It overlies the styloid process of radius. Here the radial nerve becomes subcutaneous and majority of nerve fibres can be reached in the anatomical snuff box.

A needle is inserted close to the tendon of extensor pollicis longus over the styloid process of radius and then directed towards ulnar border of wrist across the dorsum of the wrist upto the ulnar styloid process. The local anaesthetic solution 5 to 10 ml is injected across the dorsum of the wrist. About 3 ml of the local anaesthetic solution is also deposited lateral to the radial artery after aspiration test for blood.

As the branches of the radial nerve are small and numerous, block may be performed easily by a circle of subcutaneous injection (bracelet) of the local anaesthetic solution.

For analgesia of the hand (palm, web and dorsum), a median nerve block, an ulnar nerve block and a subcutaneous infiltration across dorsum of wrist to block branches of radial nerve are often satisfactory.

## Digital Nerve Block

Digital nerve block can be performed in different approaches such as metacarpal, classical and web space approaches. Never use local anaesthetic solutions which contain vasoconstrictors like adrenaline to avoid ischaemia of the digits.

### *Metacarpal Block*

The hand is kept pronated and the intermetacarpal spaces are identified. Their midpoints are located. A needle is inserted perpendicular to skin and directed vertically towards the palmar side. A finger should be placed beneath the space on the palmar side. One should be careful not to pierce the palmar aponeurosis.

The local anaesthetic solution about 2 ml is injected at the aponeurosis, another 2 ml is injected as needle is withdrawn and another 2 ml at the level of posterior border of metacarpal.

The technique is mostly painful and is indicated only when the deeper structures of the hand need to be anaesthetised.

### Classical Digital Block

The hand should be kept in prone position. The metacarpophalangeal joints are identified. A needle is inserted perpendicular to skin just distal to the joint. A finger on the palmar side should guard the direction of the needle. The needle is advanced towards the palmar border of the phalanx and the anaesthetic solution 2 to 5 ml is injected.

### Web Space Block

The appropriate web spaces are identified. A needle is inserted into the webspace in the horizontal plane and advanced to reach the metacarpophalangeal joint. After negative aspiration test for blood, the anaesthetic solution of about 5 ml should be injected slowly.

## BLOCKS OF LOWER LIMB

### Lumbar Plexus (Fig. 8.28)

The lumbar plexus is formed by the anterior primary rami of the first four lumbar nerves. It is situated in front of the transverse processes of the lumbar vertebrae. A branch from the fourth lumbar nerve joins with the fifth lumbar nerve to form the lumbosacral trunk which unties the sacral plexus. It combines in a series of loops within the psoas major muscle. The important branches of the lumbar plexus are as follows:

1. Iliohypogastric nerve $L_1$
2. Ilioinguinal nerve $T_{12}$, $L_1$
3. Genitofemoral nerve $L_1$, $L_2$
4. Femoral nerve $L_2$, $L_3$, $L_4$
5. Lateral cutaneous nerve of thigh $L_2$, $L_3$
6. Obturator nerve $L_2$, $L_3$, $L_4$

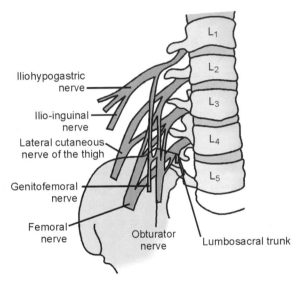

**Fig. 8.28:** Lumbar plexus

The iliohypogastric, ilioinguinal and genitofemoral nerves innervate the lower abdomen and the some upper part of lower limb. The femoral nerve, lateral cutaneous nerve of thigh and obturator nerve give sensory supply and deeper structures of the lower limb above the knee. Saphenous nerve, the terminal branch of femoral nerve gives sensory supply below the knee joint.

The lumbar plexus is usually blocked by lumbar paravertebral block (discussed earlier) and the psoas compartment block which blocks the loops of the plexus. Inguinal paravascular block can also be done.

### Lumbar Plexus Block (Psoas Compartment Block)

The patient should lie in prone position with a pillow under the abdomen. The upper edge of the $L_3$ spine is identified. A skin wheal is performed about 4 cm laterally. A long needle is inserted perpendicular to skin and advanced to contact the bony transverse process. Then the needle is little withdrawn and directed upwards in a plane parallel to midline for about 2 cm beyond the transverse process. A loss of resistance test to air from a syringe may confirm the exact location of the needle in psoas compartment in the belly of the psoas muscle.

After negative aspiration test for blood, the local anaesthetic solution 20-25 ml can be deposited.

Psoas compartment block can also be done by using the landmark at $L_4$ $L_5$ for needle insertion.

### Inguinal Paravascular Technique of Lumbar Plexus Block

Here the femoral, obturator and lateral femoral cutaneous nerves are blockd with a single injection. Thus, the technique is also known as **Three in one block.**

A fascial envelope surrounds the femoral nerve and it acts as a conduit for spreading the anaesthetic solution to block the lumbar plexus. Here the injection is given below the inguinal ligament cephalad to the site of formation of the plexus.

## Femoral Nerve Block

The femoral nerve is the largest branch of lumbar plexus derived from the posterior division of $L_2$ $L_3$ and $L_4$ nerves and descends through the psoas major muscle. It passes deep to the inguinal ligament just lateral to the femoral artery to enter the leg. It gives two divisions, anterior and posterior. The anterior division innervates the anterior and medial aspects of the thigh including the skin of the knee joint through two cutaneous nerves. It ends as saphenous nerve. The femoral nerve lies in its own fascial sheath.

### *Technique*

The patient is placed supine. The midpoint of the inguinal ligament is located. The femoral artery is palpated below the inguinal ligament. A skin wheal is made 2 to 3 cm below midinguinal point to the outer side of femoral artery. A line drawn from the anterior superior iliac spine to the symphysis pubis will indicate the inguinal ligament. The structures below the inguinal ligament are as follows from lateral to medial; nerve, artery, vein, empty space and lacunar ligament.

A needle is inserted perpendicular to skin lateral to femoral artery. After negative aspiration test for blood, 5 to 10 ml of anaesthetic solution is deposited. Paraesthesia may be obtained.

## Block of Lateral Femoral Cutaneous Nerve

It is derived from posterior divisions of $L_2$ and $L_3$ nerves. It emerges behind the psoas major muscle, crosses the pelvis and passes deep to the inguinal ligament to enter the leg. It supplies the skin of anterolateral aspects of thigh as far as the knee anteriorly.

The block is usually done along with other blocks (femoral, sciatic, obturator) for operative procedures on or above the knee joint. It may be used for pain relief due to fascia lata pain, neuralgia of thigh etc.

## Technique

The patient is placed supine. Anterior superior iliac spine and the inguinal ligament are located. A skin wheal is made 2 to 3 cm medial to anterior superior iliac spine and just superior to inguinal ligament. A needle is inserted through the wheal perpendicular to skin and advanced gently to touch the iliac bone. About 5 to 10 ml the local anaesthetic solution is deposited after negative aspiration test. The needle is then little withdrawn and directed 2 to 3 cm inferiorly or just below the inguinal ligament. About 5 to 10 ml of the solution is injected there.

## Obturator Nerve Block

The obturator nerve is derived from lumbar plexus arising from anterior divisions of $L_2$, $L_3$ and $L_4$ nerves. It divides into anterior and posterior branches. Besides their motor supply the anterior branch supplies sensory fibres to the hip joint and medial aspect of thigh and the posterior branch sends a branch to knee joint. A cutaneous nerve supplies a variable area on the lateral aspect of thigh.

The block may be *indicated* for procedures involving the knee joint and medial aspect of thigh. It is also indicated to relieve painful hip joint, adductor muscle spasm, etc. It may be needed to supplement sciatic, femoral and lateral femoral cutaneous nerve blocks for surgery on or above the knee joint.

## Technique

The block can be performed in the obturator canal below the superior ramus of the pubis between pectineus and the obturator externus.

The patient is placed supine. The pubic tubercle is located. A skin wheal is made 2 cm below and lateral to pubic tubercle. A needle is inserted through the wheal perpendicular to skin and advanced to touth the bone at about 3 to 5 cm deep. This is usually the inferior or horizontal ramus of the pubic bone. It is little withdrawn and redirected cephalad and laterally to slide off the pubis into the obturator foramen.

After negative aspiration test 10 to 15 ml of local anaesthetic solution is deposited. Successful block causes paresis of adductor muscles.

## Sciatic Nerve Block (Figs 8.29 and 8.30)

The sacral plexus is formed by the lumbosacral trunk of the lumbar plexus ($L_4$ and $L_5$) and anterior primary ramus of $S_1$ and part of $S_2$ and $S_3$ nerves. These nerves converge and gives rise to sciatic nerve. It is about 2 cm wide as it leaves the pelvis. It is the largest nerve in the body.

The nerve divides into common peroneal and the tibial nerves usually on the backside of midthigh. The sciatic nerve gives articular branches to hip joint and motor supply to hamstring muscles. The tibial nerve gives articular branches to the knee and ankle joints and muscular supply to the calf muscles and the plantar muscles of the foot. The peroneal nerve gives sensory supply to the proximal lateral area of lower leg and the dorsum foot and articular supply to knee.

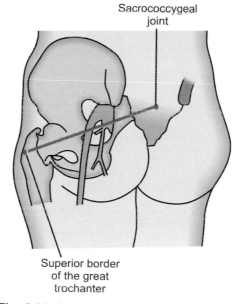

**Fig. 8.29:** Landmarks of sciatic nerve block

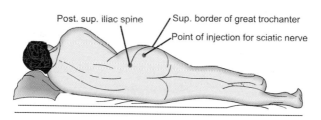

**Fig. 8.30:** Landmarks of sciatic nerve block

The nerve leaves the pelvis through the greater sciatic foramen below the pyriformis muscle and after that the nerve lies on the spine of ischium.

## *Classical Sciatic Nerve Block (Figs 8.31 and 8.32)*

The patient is placed in lateral position with the side to be blocked up and slightly rolled forward. The bottom leg is extended and straight and top leg bent at 90° at the knee and hip (Sim's position).

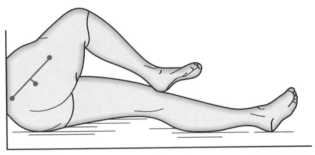

**Fig. 8.31:** Sciatic nerve block (posterior approach). 1. Posterior superior iliac spine; 2. Greater trochanter; 3. Site for injection

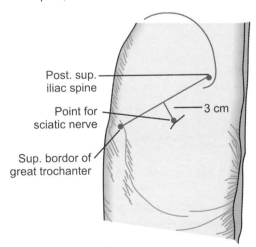

**Fig. 8.32:** Sciatic nerve location

The posterior superior iliac spine and greater trochanter of the femur are identified. These two points are joined by a line and its midpoint is located. A skin wheal is made about 5 cm below perpendicular to the line where it intersects a line between greater trochanter and the distal sacrum. It landmarks the ischial spine and sciatic nerve.

A 10 cm needle is inserted through the wheal perpendicular to skin and advanced to reach the nerve to elicit paraesthesia. If it touches the bone (posterior wall of ilium) the needle should be directed medially until it slides off the bone into sciatic notch. If the nerve is touched, the needle should be little withdrawn to avoid intraneural injection. About 25 ml of 1.5% lignocaine or 0.5% bupivacaine is injected to produce the block.

### Anterior Approach for Sciatic Nerve Block (Fig. 8.33)

The patient is positioned supine. A line is drawn along the inguinal ligament from the anterior superior iliac spine to the pubic tubercle. The line is divided in three equal parts. The junction of the medial and middle parts is located. From that point a perpendicular line is extended inferiorly and laterally.

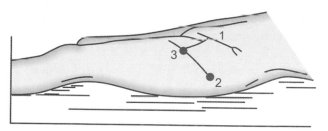

**Fig. 8.33:** Sciatic nerve block (anterior approach). 1.Inguinal ligament; 2. Greater trochanter; 3. Site for injection

Another line is drawn parallel to the first line starting at the greater trochanter of femur. The interaction of this line with the perpendicular line is the point of needle insertion.

A skin wheal is raised and a long 15 cm needle is inserted through the wheal perpendicular to skin. It is advanced gently to touch the bone. It is slightly withdrawn and redirected medially to walk off the bone and advanced further for about 5 cm. Paraesthesia may be elicited. Nerve stimulator may help to locate the nerve position. After aspiration 20 to 30 ml of local anaesthetic solution is injected.

### *Lithotomy Approach for Sciatic Nerve Block*

The patient is placed supine and one assistant should hold the leg to be blocked in lithotomy position with knee and hip flexed to 90°. A line is drawn from greater trochanter and ischial tuberosity. A skin wheal is raised 1 cm above the midpoint of the line. A long needle is inserted through the wheal perpendicular to skin. The needle is advanced to pass through the muscles and intermuscular septum towards the nerve. If it touches the bone, the needle is reangled medially to place the needle tip medial to lesser trochanter. Paraesthesia may be obtained. Nerve stimulator may help to locate the nerve. Following proper location of the nerve about 10 ml of the local anaesthetic solution is injected.

The technique is rather simple and can be done easily. But positioning may be difficult in presence of painful joints. An assistant is always needed for proper positioning.

### Popliteal Fossa Block (Fig. 8.34)

The two terminal branches of the sciatic nerve can be easily blocked while passing through the popliteal fossa at the back of the knee joint. The apex of the popliteal space is bounded by hamstring muscles, the biceps femoris on the lateral side, semimembranosus and semitendinosus on medial side and the popliteal muscle forms the floor.

The tibial branch runs through the middle of fossa and then along the back of the leg to the space between medial malleolus and the heel. Then it divides into the medial and lateral plantar nerves. At the ankle the nerve is known as posterior tibial nerve.

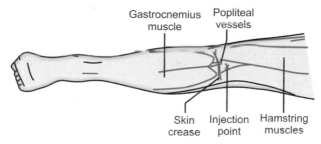

**Fig. 8.34:** Popliteal fossa block

*Technique*

The patient is placed prone and the popliteal fossa is outlined from the tendinous hamstrings above and origin of gastrocnemius muscle heads below. Posterior skin crease (line of bend of the knee) is identified. This is the widest part of the popliteal fossa. A little flexion of knee joint helps to feel the pulsation of popliteal artery.

A skin wheal is raised just lateral to the pulsation and 2 to 3 cm above the skin crease. A needle is inserted through the wheal perpendicular to skin and advanced 3 to 4 cm deep. Paraesthesia may be obtained, if the nerve is touched. A nerve stimulator may be helpful to note the correct positioning. Aspiration test for blood should be done. About 10 to 15 ml of the local anaesthetic solution should be injected gently. Care should be taken to avoid intravascular injection. Lignocaine 1.5% or bupivacaine 0.5% solution can be used.

## Saphenous Nerve Block (Figs 8.35 and 8.36)

The patient is placed in supine position. The leg is externally rotated. The medial epicondyle of tibia is located. A skin wheal is made about 2 cm posteromedial to the tibial tuberosity. A needle is inserted through the wheal in the subcutaneous plane and about 10 ml of the local anaesthetic solution is injected as it is advanced towards the posterior of the condyle.

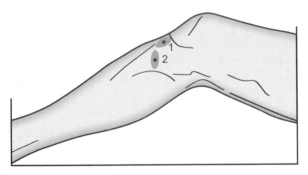

**Fig. 8.35:** Saphenous nerve block at knee at the medial side of the tibial tuberosity. 1. Tibial tuberosity; 2. Subcut. infiltration

The saphenous nerve can also blocked at the distal part in the *ankle joint*. Here also the patient is placed supine and the leg externally rotated. The long saphenous vein is located near the ankle. A skin wheal is made 1 cm proximal and 1 cm anterior to medial malleolus and about 3 to 5 ml of the

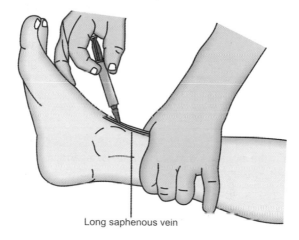
Long saphenous vein

**Fig. 8.36:** Saphenous nerve block at ankle. Injection site between medial malleolus and long saphenous vein

local anaesthetic solution is infiltrated subcutaneously around the vein. Care should be taken to avoid intravascular injection.

## Peroneal Nerve Block (Fig. 8.37)

The common peroneal nerve can be blocked near the knee joint. The patient is placed supine. The head of the fibula is palpated. Here the common peroneal nerve crosses the fibula and is usually palpable just 2 to 4 cm below the head. About 5 ml of the local anaesthetic solution is injected.

## Tibial Nerve Block at Knee (Fig. 8.38)

Tibial nerve can be blocked at knee. The lateral and medial epicondyles of femur are identified while the leg is pronated. A line is joined between the two. The needle is inserted in the

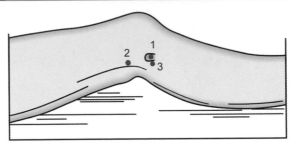

**Fig. 8.37:** Common peroneal nerve block (2 cm below head of fibula is the site). 1. Head of fibula; 2. Biceps femoris tendon; 3. Site for injection

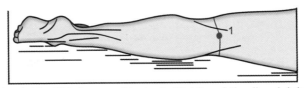

**Fig. 8.38:** Tibial nerve block. 1. Middle of the line joining lateral and medial condyle of femur

middle of the line vertical to skin about 3 cm deep and the injection is given.

### Block of Deep Peroneal Nerve at Ankle (Figs 8.39 and 8.40)

The deep peroneal nerve and superficial peroneal nerve are the branches of common peroneal nerve. These two nerves are usually blocked in combination to provide good anaesthesia for foot operation.

The patient is in supine position. A line is drawn through the two malleoli. It usually corresponds the natural skin crease on the dorsal aspect of the foot. The dorsalis pedis artery

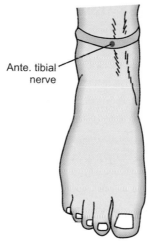

**Fig. 8.39:** Anterior tibial nerve block at ankle

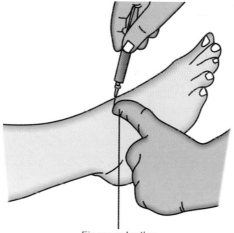

**Fig. 8.40:** Deep peroneal nerve block at ankle

pulsation is felt at this level between the extensor hallucis longus medially and extensor digitorum longus laterally. A skin wheal is raised just medial to pulsation. Then a needle is inserted through the wheal for about 1 cm forward. It may touch the bone. Then it should be little withdrawn and reangled. About 5 ml of the local anaesthetic solution should be deposited. Intravascular injection and/or tendon injury should be avoided.

***Superficial peroneal nerve block*** can also be done along with deep peroneal block at ankle. After completion of the block the needle is withdrawn in the subcutaneous tissue and reangled laterally. About 7 ml of the local anaesthetic solution is injected along the line joining the two malleoli (Fig. 8.41).

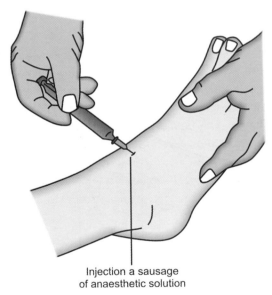

Injection a sausage
of anaesthetic solution

**Fig. 8.41:** Superficial peroneal nerve block at ankle

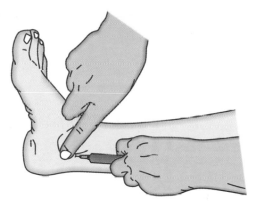

**Fig. 8.42:** Posterior tibial nerve block

## Posterior Tibial Nerve Block at Ankle (Figs 8.42 and 8.43)

The patient is positioned supine with the leg to be anaesthetised crossing the knee. The pulsation of the posterior tibial artery is felt and a finger is kept at that point. A needle is inserted at a point just behind the medial malleolus in a plane parallel to tibia. The needle is gently advanced towards the palpating finger deep to the pulsation of the posterior tibial artery. Paraesthesia may be obtained and about 5 ml of the local anaesthetic solution may be injected after negative aspiration test for blood. Take care not to inject subperiosteally.

## Foot Block (Fig. 8.44)

It is indicated for all operations of foot and toes. Medial malleolus and tibial artery are identified. Tibial nerve block is done on both sides of tibial artery. Subcutaneous infiltration is made above the medial malleolus to block saphenous nerve.

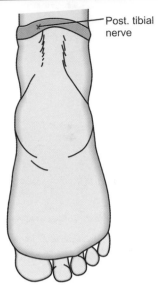

**Fig. 8.43:** Posterior tibial nerve block

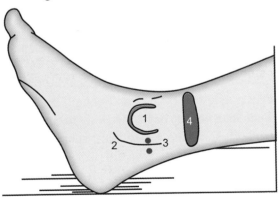

**Fig. 8.44:** Foot block. Tibial nerve and saphenous nerve block at ankle. 1. Medial malleolus; 2. Tibial ankle; 3. Injection sites for tibial nerve block; 4. Subcut. infiltration for saphenous nerve block

The nerve can also be blocked deep to the sustentaculum tali which is a ridge of bone about 1 cm distal to the medial malleolus. At that point the needle is inserted to pierce the flexor retinaculum. This may be felt as loss of resistance and about 6 ml of the local anaesthetic solution is deposited.

## Sural Nerve Block

The sural nerve may be blocked in the groove between the lateral malleous and calcaneum.

The patient is positioned supine with the foot to be anaesthetised inverted. A needle is inserted behind the lateral malleolus and directed towards the lateral border of Achiles tendon. About 5 ml of the local anaesthetic solution is injected and some solution is also injected subcutaneously between the lateral malleolus and Achiles tendon.

## Digital Nerve Block

### *Metatarsal Block (Fig. 8.45)*

Metatarsal block may be indicated for anaesthesia of the intrinsic muscles and deeper structures of the forefoot.

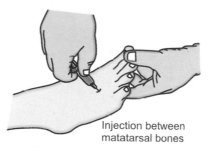

Injection between
matatarsal bones

**Fig. 8.45:** Metatarsal block

The spaces between the metatarsal bones are carefully identified. A needle is inserted into the space vertically downwards towards the plantar surface upto half way between the dorsum and plantar surface. A finger may be placed on the sole to guide. Care should be taken not to pierce the plantar fascia. About 2 ml of the local anaesthetic solution is injected and a further infiltration should be done while withdrawing the needle.

Digital nerve block (Fig. 8.46) can also be done at the level of metatarsophalangeal joints on either side of the toes. The needle is inserted just distal to the metatarsophalangeal joint above the web space vertically downwards to inject about 3 ml of the local anaesthetic solution. Here the analgesia of the toes alone is obtained.

Digital nerve block can also be done at the web space of the toes. A needle is inserted into the web space and the needle point is directed to the metatarsophalangeal joint. About 4 ml of the local anaesthetic solution should be deposited (Fig. 8.47).

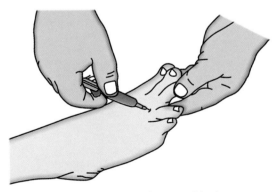

**Fig. 8.46:** Digital nerve block

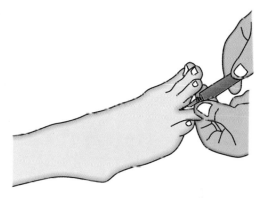

**Fig. 8.47·** Web space block

- No vasconstrictors like adrenaline should be used with the local anaesthetic solution in cases of digital nerve blocks, otherwise ischaemia may occur and it may be dangerous.

# CHAPTER 9

# Miscellaneous

# RETROBULBAR BLOCK (FIG. 9.1)
# (PINNOCK ET AL 1996)

Retrobulbar block is an important regional anaesthesia technique for intraocular surgery. It produces effective sensory and motor block (akinesia) and is mostly reliable. It is often combined with a facial nerve block which produces paralysis of the orbicularis oculi. The retrobulbar block affects mainly the ciliary ganglion and the long and short ciliary nerves. The injection is given to a point behind the eye near the apex of orbit where the ciliary ganglion lies just within the muscle cone.

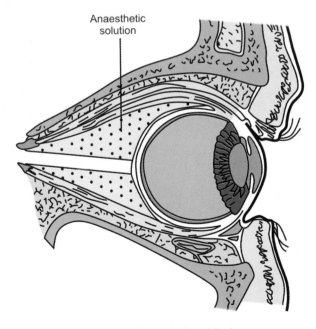

Anaesthetic
solution

**Fig. 9.1:** Retrobulbar block

## Technique

The patient is placed in supine position. The cornea and conjunctiva are topically anaesthetised with two drops of local anaesthetic solution over the cornea.

The patient is asked to look straight forward. A needle is inserted through the reflection of conjunctiva below the lateral limbus and gently advanced parallel to the floor of the orbit in a depth for about 15 mm. Then the needle tip is redirected slightly medially and upwards to enter the muscle cone usually at a depth of about 30 mm. After negative aspiration test, 3 to 5 ml of the local anaesthetic solution (2% lignocaine or 0.75% bupivacaine) is injected. Care must be taken not to injure the globe by the needle. In such cases the patient may feel severe pain and the globe deviates suddenly. The needle should be withdrawn and redirected.

The onset time for the anaesthesia block is usually within 5 minutes. But its failure rate is less than 1% in skilled hands.

## Complications

1. Retrobulbar haemorrhage.
2. Intravascular injection.
3. Systemic toxicity, convulsion.
4. Intraneural injection.
5. Injury to globe.
6. Central retinal occlusion.
7. Subdural or subarachnoid injection.
8. Oculocardiac reflex.

## PERIBULBAR BLOCK (FIG. 9.2)
## (PINNOCK ET AL 1996)

It is a good alternative to retrobulbar block and is associated with only few complications. It is performed by injecting the local anaesthetic solution around the eye and not in the eye's muscle cone.

The patient is placed supine and topical anaesthesia with 2 drops of local anaesthetic solution over the cornea and conjunctiva is performed. The patient is asked to lie their gaze straight ahead. A needle is inserted through the conjunctival reflection below the lateral limbus vertically. Then it is advanced

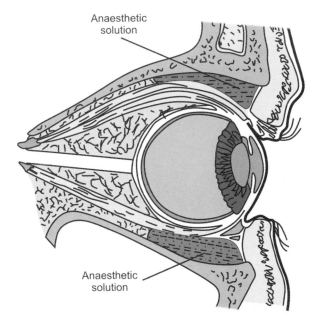

**Fig. 9.2:** Peribulbar block

parallel to the floor of orbit and tangential to globe to place the needle point outside the muscle cone. After negative aspiration for blood, about 10 ml of the local anaesthetic solution is injected gently. If the needle point touches the bone, it should be realigned.

A second injection of about 5 ml anaesthetic solution may be needed through the conjunctiva in the medial canthus medial to the caruncle. The needle is inserted parallel to the medial wall of the orbit and advanced to reach outside the muscle cone. Aspiration test must be done before injection.

The failure rate of peribulbar block is usually high about 10% and its onset time is about 10 minutes. But the incidence of serious complications is low.

### Disadvantages

1. Requires at least two injections.
2. Requires large volume of anaesthetic.
3. Onset time is longer.

### Advantages

1. Low incidence of serious complications.
2. Separate facial nerve block is not needed in peribulbar block as the large volume of the anaesthetic solution penetrates the eyelids directly.

## FACIAL NERVE BLOCK

It is often needed to supplement retrobulbar block. A skin wheal is raised 1 cm lateral to the lateral margin of the orbit on the side to be anaesthetised. A needle is inserted downwards to the periosteum and about 2 ml of anaesthetic solution is injected. The needle is then reangled towards the cheek bone prominence and about 2 ml of anaesthetic solution is injected. The needle is then withdrawn to the skin wheal and is advanced cephalad to inject another 2 ml solution. Temporal and zygomatic branches of the facial nerve are blocked.

Alternatively, the entire facial nerve can be blocked at the temporomandibular joint. But it is usually not needed in eye surgery.

## TOPICAL ANALGESIA OF THE NASAL CAVITIES

1. Lignocaine 1.5% with adrenaline may be used for this purpose. The patient is positioned supine with the head and neck hyperextended and about 20 ml of the anaesthetic solution is poured in one nostril. The patient is asked to breathe through the mouth. This is repeated in the other nostril also. After 2 to 3 minutes the patient is asked to sit up and blow through nose. The patient should not swallow the solution and is asked to spit it out. The whole nasal mucosa becomes anaesthetised.
2. The nasal cavities can be sprayed with 4% lignocaine. The excess solution should be rejected and not swallowed.
3. The nasal cavity may be packed with a rollar gauze soaked with the local anaesthetic solution. Adrenaline may also be combined to provide the ischaemic field.

## TOPICAL ANALGESIA OF LARYNX

Here a laryngeal spray is used to administer a fine mist of the local anaesthetic solution on the mucosa of the larynx and upper trachea. Lignocaine 4% solution gives satisfactory analgesia. It minimises the autonomic reflexes and circulatory changes associated with endotracheal intubation.

## TRANSTRACHEAL TECHNIQUE OF TOPICAL ANAESTHESIA (FIG. 9.3)

The patient is positioned supine with head hyperextended. He is asked not to cough, talk or swallow when the needle is in place.

The thyroid and cricoid cartilage are identified on the neck of the patient. The space between the two is known as cricothyroid membrane.

With proper aseptic precautions and preparations, a skin wheal is made over the cricothyroid membrane. A needle with an attached 2 ml syringe filled with a topically effective

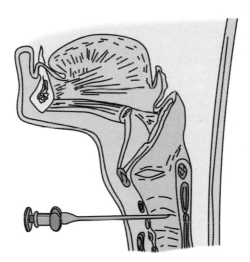

**Fig. 9.3:** Transtracheal technique of topical anaesthesia

anaesthetic like lignocaine 4% is inserted in the midline perpendicular to skin through the cricothyroid membrane. It is advanced until lack of resistance is felt. It then indicates the intratracheal position. This may be confirmed by aspirating of air. Then the solution is injected quickly and the needle is withdrawn. The patient is asked to cough vigorously to spread the solution.

The mouth, pharynx and supraglottic area may be sprayed with lignocaine for further anaesthesia. The piriform fossae are made insensitive by application of swabs soaked in the local anaesthetic solution with the help of Magill forceps.

## TOPICAL ANALGESIA FOR BRONCHOSCOPY

Regional analgesia may be preferred as it is safer than general anaesthesia particularly when there is excessive secretion, airway disturbances and low general condition of the patient.

1. The gums, tongue and pharynx may be sprayed with 4% lignocaine solution. Lignocaine viscous 2% solution may be swallowed.
2. The piriform fossae are made insensitive by application cotton pledgets soaked in the local anaesthetic solution with the Magill forceps.
3. Trachea may be anaesthetised by transtracheal injection of 2 to 3 ml of 4% lignocaine solution through a needle inserted in cricothyroid membrane. Complications of transtracheal injection may include infection, broken needle, surgical emphysema, etc.

After topical analgesia the patient should be instructed not to eat or drink for at least 3 hours or until the protective reflexes return.

- *Note:*

Nerves involved in topical analgesia for endotracheal intubation.

A. *Tongue:*
  1. Sensory of anterior two-third: Lingual branch of mandibular nerve.
  2. Taste of anterior two-third: Chorda tympani of facial nerve.
  3. Base and sides, both sensation and taste: Lingual branch of glossopharyngeal nerve.
  4. Root of tongue: Superior laryngeal nerve.

B. *Pharynx:* Pharyngeal plexus (Glossopharyngeal, vagus and sympathetics).

C. *Larynx:*
  1. Superior laryngeal nerve.
  2. Recurrent laryngeal nerve.

D. *Trachea:* Vagus, recurrent laryngeal nerve and sympathetics.

## LOCAL INFILTRATION FOR DENTAL EXTRACTION

The patient is usually on supine position on a dental chair. The appropriate tooth should be identified. A needle is inserted at the junction of adherent mucoperiosteum of gum with the free mucous membrane of the cheek and advanced parallel to the long axis of the tooth. About 1 ml of 2% lignocaine solution with adrenaline is injected gently superficial to the periosteum on the buccal and either the lingual or palatal side. Extraction of tooth should be done at least after 5 minutes of injection. Before extraction, analgesic effect must be tested.

The technique is mostly satisfactory for all teeth except the lower molars.

## TOPICAL ANALGESIA OF THE URETHRA

Lignocaine jelly 2% is available in tubes along with a plastic nozzle. It can be used for topical analgesia of the urethra indicated for difficult catheterisation, urethral dilatation, instrumentation, etc. Full aseptic measures should be taken.

The sterilized nozzle is introduced through the urethral orifice and the tube is squeezed inside the urethra. About 10 ml of the lignocaine jelly is given. After withdrawal of the nozzle the penis is clamped and the drug is gently massaged into the posterior urethra. Analgesia occurs within 10 to 15 minutes after which the instrumentation can be done satisfactorily. Care should be taken not to exceed the safe maximum dose.

## FIELD BLOCK FOR CIRCUMCISION

Penis gets sensory supply from the terminal branches of pudendal nerves, the dorsal nerves of penis, one on each side of the midline against the dorsal surface of the corpus cavernosum. The skin of the base of penis is supplied by ilioinguinal and genitofemoral nerves. The posterior scrotal branches of perineal nerves pass paraurethrally to the ventral surface and frenum of penis.

A subcutaneous ring wheal is performed at the base of the penis. The dorsal nerve is blocked on each side by injecting the anaesthetic solution into the dorsum of the penis at the corpus cavernosum. Then the penis is pulled upwards and the anaesthetic solution is injected near the base of penis into the groove between cavernosa and the corpus spongiosum. It blocks the paraurethral scrotal nerves.

- Adrenaline must not be used in anaesthetic solution as it may cause ischaemic necrosis as the arteries of penis are end arteries.

## REGIONAL REFRIGERATION ANAESTHESIA

The application of cold to a localised part of the body can produce a local nerve block. When skin temperature is maintained at about 8°C for about 3 hours, the cold penetrates to all depths and the part becomes insensitive. In poor risk, malnourished patients particularly in rapidly spreading gangrene and sepsis cases, the technique was used for amputation surgery. Amputation of leg in arteriosclerotic or diabetic gangrene can also be done. It can also be used for operations on the fingers, toes, hands and wrist. But the technique is cumbersome and fussy and is not used nowadays.

### Technique

Ice bags are applied to the limb for about 30 minutes before applying the tourniquet. The tourniquet is applied to occlude the circulation about 4 inches above the site of operation.

The limb is covered with cracked ice. The ice may be encased with rubber sheet and water should be drained properly. The skin temperature should be maintained about 8° to 10°C.

Time of refrizeration will vary according to the site of operation and bulk of tissue. It is usually as follows: thigh 2-5 hours; upper leg 2 hours, lower leg 1 hour and foot 1 hour, for arm 2 hours, for hand 1 hour and for fingers and toes 30 minutes.

After completion of refrizeration the limb should be dried. The surgical team should be directed to operate as quickly as possible. Warm object should not be used. Cold instruments should be used. The tourniquet should be removed after the end of operation. Amputation stump may be packed in ice bags for 24 to 48 hours.

### Advantages

1. Mortality rate is low.
2. Postoperative analgesia.
3. Absence of shock, less blood loss.
4. Metabolic responses to injury less.
5. Less chance of wound infection.

### Disadvantages

1. Cumbersome technique.
2. Delayed healing.
3. Time consuming.
4. Loose tourniquet may cause failure.

## THERAPEUTIC NERVE BLOCKS

Therapeutinc nerve blocks are usually done with local anaesthetics, neurolytics or neuraxial placement of opioid.

Nerve blocks with local anaesthetics alleviate chronic pain in various ways.

1. Interruption of sensory pathways of pain.
2. Nerve blocks may prevent the onset of self-perpeturating pain syndromes such as phantom limb, sympathetically maintained pain syndromes.

3. Nerve block aids physiotherapy, manipulation, etc.
4. Steroids added in local anaesthetic may provide long-term antiinflammatory effects.
5. Sympathetic block in sympathetically maintained pain. In patients with vascular disease the vascular supply of an ischaemic area can be improved.

## NEUROLYTIC BLOCKS

Neurolytic block with either alcohol or phenol can produce long lasting relief particularly in cancer patients. Neurolytic agents like alcohol or phenol directly destroy neural tissue and these must be deposited close to the peripheral nerves or into the subarachnoid or epidural space. But their effects are not permanent and may last from days to months, so it may have to be repeated.

Phenol is used as 5 to 10% strength and it is hyperbaric. It produces local anaesthetic effect and causes no pain on injection.

Ethyl alcohol is used as 50 to 100% concentration and it is hypobaric. It has no local anaesthetic effect and causes pain on injection.

Motor deficits or a denervation hypersensitivity type of pain may occur and may be difficult to treat. Thus, neurolytic drugs should be better used in subarachnoid or epidural space. Destructive nerve blocks should be restricted for patients with cancer with a short life expectancy and it is better avoided in chronic nonmalignant pain. Extreme caution is needed to needle placement and to restrict extent of spread of the neurolytic agent and thus fluoroscopy is mostly helpful.

## DIAGNOSTIC AND THERAPEUTIC NERVE BLOCKS

1. Subarachnoid block
2. Epidural / extradural block
3. Trigeminal nerve block
4. Stellate ganglion block
5. Brachial plexus block
6. Intercostal nerve block
7. Lumbar sympathetic block
8. Coeliac plexus block
9. Intravenous regional neural block.

## NEURAXIAL OPIOIDS

Chronic pain syndromes particularly due to cancer are being satisfactorily managed by neuraxial (subarachnoid or extradural) administration of opioids. Morphine is being widely used for this purpose. For long-term therapy subarachnoid or epidural catheters can be implanted. The catheter can be kept for indefinite period. Implanted infusion device can also be used. The device includes a percutaneously refillable reservoir for opioid and a pumping device to administer the drug through the catheter inside in subarachnoid / epidural space.

### Advantages

1. Satisfactory pain relief
2. Prolonged pain relief, limitless in catheter technique
3. Absence of sympathetic block
4. Absence of skeletal muscle paralysis
5. Respiratory depression delayed and less.

6. Less incidence of side effects like pruritus, sedation, urinary retention, nausea/vomiting.

## Disadvantages

1. Need for skilled anaesthetist to perform the technique and monitor.
2. Tolerance to opioid can occur in some cases.
3. Abrupt discontinuance of neuraxial opioid administration may lead to opioid withdrawal syndrome.
4. Problems of catheterisation such as leakage, occlusion, infection, etc. may occur.

## CONTINUOUS CATHETER TECHNIQUES OF NERVE BLOCKS

The duration of peripheral nerve block from single injection of the local anaesthetic drug usually ranges from 2 to 12 hours depending upon the drug, its strength and volume and the nature of nerve. Many times prolonged effect is needed for better patient care as in cases of major surgical procedures, reconstructive procedures, chronic pain syndromes, in management of cancer pain and so on. These cases may benefit with continuous catheter technique where prolonged nerve block can be effectively maintained for several days or even weeks.

The technique is mostly simple and easy to perform by introducing a sterile fine catheter into the space surrounding the appropriate nerve or plexus and administering the local anaesthetic solution either in incremental doses or continuously in a strict judicious way. The technique is mostly similar as in continuous epidural technique.

Continuous catheter technique is commonly used in some particular nerve blocks.

1. Brachial plexus block–Axillary or subclavian perivascular approach.
2. Intercostal nerve block.
3. Interpleural.
4. Paravertebral–thoracic, lumbar plexus block.
5. Sciatic nerve block.
6. Femoral nerve block.

## Advantages

1. *Prolonged analgesia*:
   (a) Postoperative pain relief following major surgery, total knee replacement, thoracic surgery.
   (b) Chronic pain syndromes: Cancer pain management. Reflex sympathetic dystrophy.
2. *Sympathetic block*:
   (a) To improve vascularity in areas of critical perfusion.
   (b) To improve the graft vascularity and to reduce the incidence of graft failure.
3. The need of narcotic drugs is reduced.
4. Active rehabilitation, joint movement, physiotherapy, limb function possible.
5. Patient's psychological status becomes better.

## Disadvantages

1. Needs skill and experience on the part of the anesthesiologist.
2. Needs monitoring during the procedure.
3. Extra care is needed.

4. Infection, obstruction, kinking, misplacement, etc. can occur as catheter problems.
5. Nerve damage is possible.

## Technique

The sterile intravenous cannula, intravenous needles, syringes, epidural needle, epidural catheter, hypodermic needles, local anaesthetic drugs, appropriate infusion set, etc. should be kept ready.

Peripheral nerve stimulator is often needed to locate the nerve properly. Final positioning of the catheter may be confirmed by the use of an image intensifier and a suitable water soluble X-ray contrast medium.

A good assistant and a skilled radiographer are mostly helpful.

Strict sterile precautions, skin preparation, draping, etc. are needed to reduce the risk infection.

The technique is mostly similar to standard technique of nerve block and to inserting a suitable catheter in the appropriate space surrounding the nerve or plexus. When the needle is correctly placed in position about 10 ml of normal saline may be injected first to open up the perineural space. This will aid the introduction of catheter easily and smoothly.

After the catheter is placed in position, it must be secured properly and sterile dressing should be applied.

## REGIONAL ANALGESIA IN NORMAL DELIVERY

Mild uterine contractions occur throughout pregnancy. These become rhythmical and coordinated in the last 2 to 3 weeks before term. In the first stage of labour these are more regular and intense to dilate the cervix. In the second stage the contractions become intense with reflex contraction of abdominal muscles and diaphragm. It helps for expulsion of foetus. Uterine contractions rapidly decrease in frequency and intensity after the expulsion of foetus in the third stage of labour.

## Nerve Supply

A. *Sensory:*
   (a) Upper uterine segment through sympathetic nerves to $T_{11}$ and $T_{12}$.
   (b) Lower uterine segment through sacral parasympathetic $S_2$, $S_3$ and $S_4$.
   (c) Birth canal through the pudendal nerve.
B. *Motor:* Uterus receives both sympathetic and parasympathetic fibres. Sympathetic fibres pass to the superior, middle and inferior hypogastric plexus, and thereafter through the uterosacral and broad ligaments of uterus. Parasympathetic fibres ($S_2$, $S_3$, $S_4$) join the sympathetic fibres in the pelvis or uterosacral ligaments.

## Role of Regional Analgesia

### Spinal Block

It can be safely used for normal delivery or mild/low forceps delivery. Block should extend to $S_1$. This block is also helpful for outlet forceps with episiotomy.

For high forceps or intrauterine manipulations spinal block should reach $T_{11}$. Prevent hypotension as it increases the risk of foetal hypoxia.

Advantages of spinal block may include no foetal respiratory depression, satisfactory relaxation of pelvic floor muscles, no risk of aspiration pneumonitis and intact consciousness during delivery.

### Epidural Block

It can be satisfactorily used either in single injection technique or a continuous catheter technique. Usually a block upto $T_{10}$ is mostly satisfactory. It paralyses the sympathetic efferent supply of uterus and aids dilatation of cervix. It should be noted that smaller than usual doses of the local anaesthetic are needed in obstetrics.

### Caudal Block

Continuous caudal block is mostly safe for the mother and baby. It causes excellent relaxation of the lower birth canal and provides good analgesia. The third stage of labour is usually short and postpartum blood loss is minimal. But one should aware of its complications such as high forceps rate, accidental subarachnoid block, infection, intrafoetal injection, and so on.

### Pudendal Nerve Block with Local Infiltration

This may be indicated for normal delivery, episiotomy, outlet forceps delivery, and repair of perineal injury. Transperineal approach is safely used. It is often helpful and safe in cases of foetal distress, delayed second stage of labour and assisted breech delivery.

## *Paracervical Nerve Block*

Here the local anaesthetic solution is injected into the loose areolar tissue at the sides of cervix to block the pain sensation from the uterus. The nerve fibres from the uterus and cervix form a plexus at the base of broad ligament and pass to the presacral nerves.

It provides satisfactory pain relief and aids cervical dilatation.

# BIBLIOGRAPHY

1. Al-Shaikh B, Stacey S. Essentials of anaesthetic equipment, New York. Churchill Livingstone, 1995.
2. Astra – IDL Ltd., Regional Anaesthesia, Bangalore.
3. Collins VJ. Principles of Anaesthesiology. Kothari Book Depot. 1972.
4. Lee JA, Alkinson RS. A synopsis of anaesthesia. Bristol. John Wright and Sons. 1990.
5. Longnecker DE, Murphy FL. Inroduction to anaesthesia. Philadelphia WB Saunders Co. 1997.
6. McGregor AL. A synopsis of surgical anatomy. Bristol. John Wright and Sons Ltd. 1983.
7. Miller RD. Anaesthesia. Vo. 1, 2 and 3. Edinbergh. Churchill Livingstone 1986.
8. Nunn JF, Utting JE, Brown BR. General anaesthesia. London. Butterworths 1988.
9. Paul AK. Essentials of Anaesthesiology. New Delhi. Jaypee Bros. 2006.
10. Paul AK. Clinical Anaestheisa. New Delhi. Jaypee Bros. 2006.
11. Paul AK. Drugs and Equipment in Anaesthetic Practice. New Delhi. Elsevier. 2004.
12. Paul AK. Fundamentals of Paediatric Anaesthesia. New Delhi. BI Publications Pvt Ltd. 2006.
13. Reed AP. Clinical cases in Anaesthesia. New York. Churchill Livingstone. 1975.
14. Smith G, Aitkenhead AR. Textbook of Anaesthesia. London. Churchill Livingstone. 1985.
15. Stoelting RK, Miller RD. Basics of Anaesthesia. New York. Churchill Livingstone. 1994.
16. Wylie ED, Churchill Davidson HC. A Practice of Anaesthesia. London. Lloyd Luke. 1988.

# INDEX

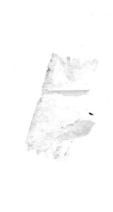